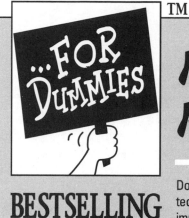
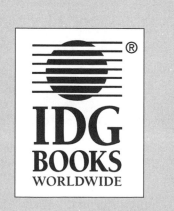

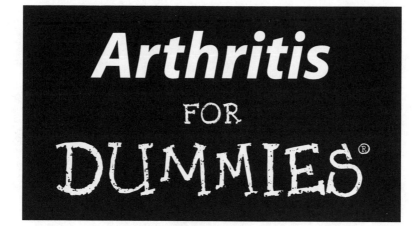

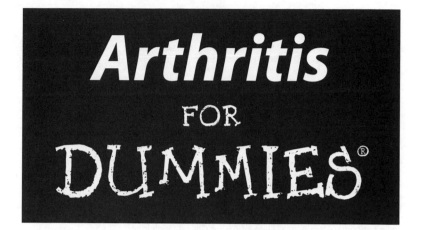

Arthritis FOR DUMMIES®

by Barry Fox and Nadine Taylor

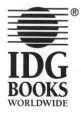

IDG Books Worldwide, Inc.
An International Data Group Company

Foster City, CA ◆ Chicago, IL ◆ Indianapolis, IN ◆ New York, NY

Arthritis For Dummies®

Published by
IDG Books Worldwide, Inc.
An International Data Group Company
919 E. Hillsdale Blvd.
Suite 400
Foster City, CA 94404
www.idgbooks.com (IDG Books Worldwide Web Site)
www.dummies.com (Dummies Press Web Site)

Library of Congress Control Number: 00-104220

ISBN: 0-7645-5258-9

Printed in the United States of America

10 9 8 7 6 5 4 3 2 1

1B/RS/QZ/QQ/IN

Distributed in the United States by IDG Books Worldwide, Inc.

Distributed by CDG Books Canada Inc. for Canada; by Transworld Publishers Limited in the United Kingdom; by IDG Norge Books for Norway; by IDG Sweden Books for Sweden; by IDG Books Australia Publishing Corporation Pty. Ltd. for Australia and New Zealand; by TransQuest Publishers Pte Ltd. for Singapore, Malaysia, Thailand, Indonesia, and Hong Kong; by Gotop Information Inc. for Taiwan; by ICG Muse, Inc. for Japan; by Intersoft for South Africa; by Eyrolles for France; by International Thomson Publishing for Germany, Austria and Switzerland; by Distribuidora Cuspide for Argentina; by LR International for Brazil; by Galileo Libros for Chile; by Ediciones ZETA S.C.R. Ltda. for Peru; by WS Computer Publishing Corporation, Inc., for the Philippines; by Contemporanea de Ediciones for Venezuela; by Express Computer Distributors for the Caribbean and West Indies; by Micronesia Media Distributor, Inc. for Micronesia; by Chips Computadoras S.A. de C.V. for Mexico; by Editorial Norma de Panama S.A. for Panama; by American Bookshops for Finland.

For general information on IDG Books Worldwide's books in the U.S., please call our Consumer Customer Service department at 800-762-2974. For reseller information, including discounts and premium sales, please call our Reseller Customer Service department at 800-434-3422.

For information on where to purchase IDG Books Worldwide's books outside the U.S., please contact our International Sales department at 317-572-3993 or fax 317-572-4002.

For consumer information on foreign language translations, please contact our Customer Service department at 1-800-434-3422, fax 317-572-4002, or e-mail rights@idgbooks.com.

For information on licensing foreign or domestic rights, please phone +1-650-653-7098.

For sales inquiries and special prices for bulk quantities, please contact our Order Services department at 800-434-4322 or write to the address above.

For information on using IDG Books Worldwide's books in the classroom or for ordering examination copies, please contact our Educational Sales department at 800-434-2086 or fax 317-572-4005.

For press review copies, author interviews, or other publicity information, please contact our Public Relations department at 650-653-7000 or fax 650-653-7500.

For authorization to photocopy items for corporate, personal, or educational use, please contact Copyright Clearance Center, 222 Rosewood Drive, Danvers, MA 01923, or fax 978-750-4470.

 is a registered trademark under exclusive license to IDG Books Worldwide, Inc., from International Data Group, Inc.

About the Authors

Barry Fox, Ph.D. and **Nadine Taylor, M.S., R.D.** are a husband-and-wife writing team living in Los Angeles, California.

Barry is the author, coauthor, or ghostwriter of numerous books, including the New York Times number one best-selling book *The Arthritis Cure* (St. Martin's, 1997). He also wrote its sequel, *Maximizing The Arthritis Cure* (St. Martin's, 1998), as well as *Syndrome X* (Simon & Schuster, 2000), *The 20/30 Fat and Fiber Diet Plan* (HarperCollins, 1999), and *Cancer Talk* (Broadway Books, 1999). Other books include *Diana and Dodi: A Love Story* (Tallfellow, 1998), *Immune For Life* (Prima Publishing, 1986), and *DLPA To End Chronic Pain and Depression* (Simon & Schuster, 1985). His books and over 160 articles covering various aspects of health, business, biography, law, and other topics have been translated into 20 languages. He is currently a Professor of Anti-Aging Studies at the University of Integrative Studies.

Nadine Taylor, M.S., R.D., a registered dietitian, penned *Green Tea* (Kensington Press, 1998), *If You Think You Have An Eating Disorder* (Dell, 1998), and *Diana and Dodi: A Love Story* (Tallfellow, 1999).

Ms. Taylor also edited the New York Times number one bestselling book *The Arthritis Cure* (St. Martin's, 1997), *To Your Health* (St. Martin's, 1997), *Foods To Heal By* (St. Martin's, 1996), and *The Healthy Prostate* (John Wiley, 1996). After a brief stint as head dietitian of the Eating Disorders Unit at Glendale Adventist Medical Center, she lectured on women's health issues to groups of health professionals throughout the country. She has also penned numerous articles on health and nutrition for the popular press.

ABOUT IDG BOOKS WORLDWIDE

Welcome to the world of IDG Books Worldwide.

IDG Books Worldwide, Inc., is a subsidiary of International Data Group, the world's largest publisher of computer-related information and the leading global provider of information services on information technology. IDG was founded more than 30 years ago by Patrick J. McGovern and now employs more than 9,000 people worldwide. IDG publishes more than 290 computer publications in over 75 countries. More than 90 million people read one or more IDG publications each month.

Launched in 1990, IDG Books Worldwide is today the #1 publisher of best-selling computer books in the United States. We are proud to have received eight awards from the Computer Press Association in recognition of editorial excellence and three from Computer Currents' First Annual Readers' Choice Awards. Our best-selling *...For Dummies®* series has more than 50 million copies in print with translations in 31 languages. IDG Books Worldwide, through a joint venture with IDG's Hi-Tech Beijing, became the first U.S. publisher to publish a computer book in the People's Republic of China. In record time, IDG Books Worldwide has become the first choice for millions of readers around the world who want to learn how to better manage their businesses.

Our mission is simple: Every one of our books is designed to bring extra value and skill-building instructions to the reader. Our books are written by experts who understand and care about our readers. The knowledge base of our editorial staff comes from years of experience in publishing, education, and journalism — experience we use to produce books to carry us into the new millennium. In short, we care about books, so we attract the best people. We devote special attention to details such as audience, interior design, use of icons, and illustrations. And because we use an efficient process of authoring, editing, and desktop publishing our books electronically, we can spend more time ensuring superior content and less time on the technicalities of making books.

You can count on our commitment to deliver high-quality books at competitive prices on topics you want to read about. At IDG Books Worldwide, we continue in the IDG tradition of delivering quality for more than 30 years. You'll find no better book on a subject than one from IDG Books Worldwide.

John Kilcullen
Chairman and CEO
IDG Books Worldwide, Inc.

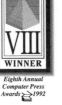

Eighth Annual Computer Press Awards 1992

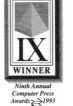

Ninth Annual Computer Press Awards 1993

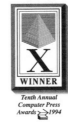

Tenth Annual Computer Press Awards 1994

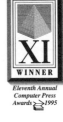

Eleventh Annual Computer Press Awards 1995

IDG is the world's leading IT media, research and exposition company. Founded in 1964, IDG had 1997 revenues of $2.05 billion and has more than 9,000 employees worldwide. IDG offers the widest range of media options that reach IT buyers in 75 countries representing 95% of worldwide IT spending. IDG's diverse product and services portfolio spans six key areas including print publishing, online publishing, expositions and conferences, market research, education and training, and global marketing services. More than 90 million people read one or more of IDG's 290 magazines and newspapers, including IDG's leading global brands — Computerworld, PC World, Network World, Macworld and the Channel World family of publications. IDG Books Worldwide is one of the fastest-growing computer book publishers in the world, with more than 700 titles in 36 languages. The "...For Dummies®" series alone has more than 50 million copies in print. IDG offers online users the largest network of technology-specific Web sites around the world through IDG.net (http://www.idg.net), which comprises more than 225 targeted Web sites in 55 countries worldwide. International Data Corporation (IDC) is the world's largest provider of information technology data, analysis and consulting, with research centers in over 41 countries and more than 400 research analysts worldwide. IDG World Expo is a leading producer of more than 168 globally branded conferences and expositions in 35 countries including E3 (Electronic Entertainment Expo), Macworld Expo, ComNet, Windows World Expo, ICE (Internet Commerce Expo), Agenda, DEMO, and Spotlight. IDG's training subsidiary, ExecuTrain, is the world's largest computer training company, with more than 230 locations worldwide and 785 training courses. IDG Marketing Services helps industry-leading IT companies build international brand recognition by developing global integrated marketing programs via IDG's print, online and exposition products worldwide. Further information about the company can be found at www.idg.com.   1/26/00

Dedication

Dedicated to Nina Ostrom Taylor, the greatest mom and mom-in-law in the world.

Authors' Acknowledgments

We'd like thank Arnold Fox, M.D., for providing us with a great deal of information on arthritis; Bernard Filner, M.D., for his careful review of our manuscript; and of course, Stacy Collins, Sherri Fugit, and the editorial staff at IDG Books Worldwide.

Publisher's Acknowledgments

We're proud of this book; please register your comments through our IDG Books Worldwide Online Registration Form located at http://my2cents.dummies.com.

Some of the people who helped bring this book to market include the following:

Acquisitions, Editorial, and Media Development

Project Editor: Sherri Fugit

Acquisitions Editor: Karen Young

Copy Editors: Donna Frederick, Billie A. Williams

Acquisitions Coordinator: Allison Solomon

Technical Editor: Dr. Bernard Filner

Editorial Managers: Kristin Cocks, Jennifer Ehrlich

Editorial Assistants: Carol Strickland, Jennifer Young

Production

Project Coordinator: Amanda Foxworth

Layout and Graphics: Amy Adrian, Jason Guy, Stephanie D. Jumper, Tracy K. Oliver, Jacque Schneider, Janet Seib, Rashell Smith, Brian Torwelle, Jeremey Unger, Erin Zeltner

Proofreaders: Laura Albert, Corey Bowen, Sally Burton, David Faust, Mary Lagu, Susan Moritz

Indexer: Southwest Indexing

Special Help
Mary Fales

General and Administrative

IDG Books Worldwide, Inc.: John Kilcullen, CEO; Bill Barry, President and COO

IDG Books Consumer Reference Group

> **Business:** Kathleen A. Welton, Vice President and Publisher; Kevin Thornton, Acquisitions Manager

> **Cooking/Gardening:** Jennifer Feldman, Associate Vice President and Publisher

> **Education/Reference:** Diane Graves Steele, Vice President and Publisher; Greg Tubach, Publishing Director

> **Lifestyles:** Kathleen Nebenhaus, Vice President and Publisher; Tracy Boggier, Managing Editor

> **Pets:** Dominique De Vito, Associate Vice President and Publisher; Tracy Boggier, Managing Editor

> **Travel:** Michael Spring, Vice President and Publisher; Suzanne Jannetta, Editorial Director; Brice Gosnell, Managing Editor

IDG Books Consumer Editorial Services: Kathleen Nebenhaus, Vice President and Publisher; Kristin A. Cocks, Editorial Director; Cindy Kitchel, Editorial Director

IDG Books Consumer Production: Debbie Stailey, Production Director

IDG Books Packaging: Marc J. Mikulich, Vice President, Brand Strategy and Research

◆

The publisher would like to give special thanks to Patrick J. McGovern, without whom this book would not have been possible.

◆

Contents at a Glance

Cartoons at a Glance

By Rich Tennant

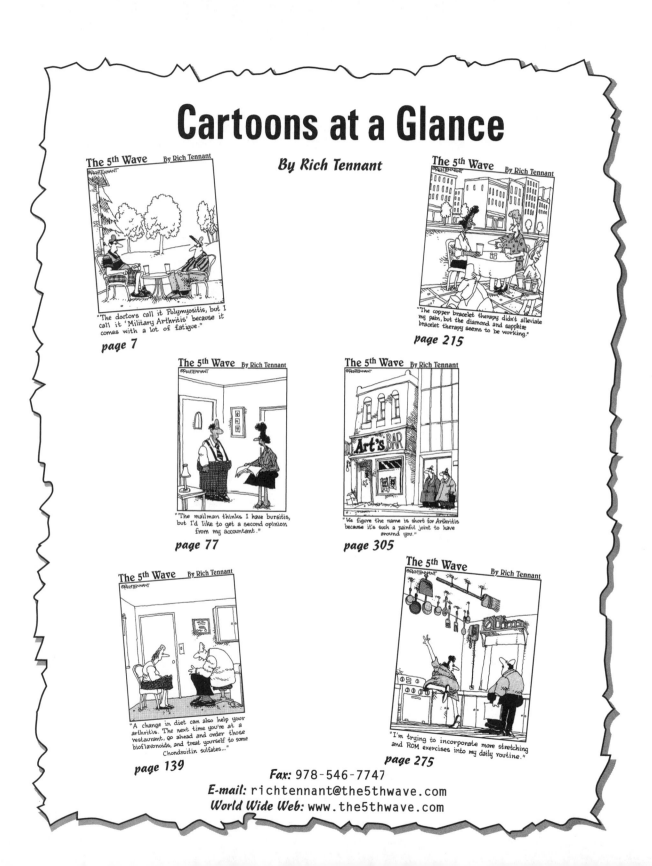

The 5th Wave By Rich Tennant

"The doctors call it Polymyositis, but I call it 'Military Arthritis' because it comes with a lot of fatigue."

page 7

The 5th Wave By Rich Tennant

"The copper bracelet therapy didn't alleviate my pain, but the diamond and sapphire bracelet therapy seems to be working."

page 215

The 5th Wave By Rich Tennant

"The mailman thinks I have bursitis, but I'd like to get a second opinion from my accountant."

page 77

The 5th Wave By Rich Tennant

Art's BAR

"We figure the name is short for Arthritis because it's such a painful joint to have around you."

page 305

The 5th Wave By Rich Tennant

"A change in diet can also help your arthritis. The next time you're at a restaurant, go ahead and order those bioflavonoids, and treat yourself to some Chondroitin sulfates..."

page 139

The 5th Wave By Rich Tennant

"I'm trying to incorporate more stretching and ROM exercises into my daily routine."

page 275

Fax: 978-546-7747
E-mail: richtennant@the5thwave.com
World Wide Web: www.the5thwave.com

Table of Contents

Introduction

● ●

*W*hether it appears as a little bit of creaky stiffness in the hip or knee or as a major case of inflammation that settles in several joints, arthritis is an unwelcome visitor that knocks on just about everybody's door sooner or later. Although there is currently no out-and-out cure for arthritis, there are many techniques for *managing* this disease — that is, controlling its symptoms so that you can get on with your life! Arthritis does *not* mean that you must spend your days relegated a rocking chair or shuffling from your bed to an easy chair and back again. Most of the time you can take charge of your disease, instead of letting it take charge of you. By following the simple techniques outlined in the this book, you can do much to control your pain, exercise away your stiffness, keep yourself on the move, and slow down or prevent progression of your disease. All it takes is a little know-how — and that's what we provide in these chapters.

About This Book

When writing this book, our goal was to provide you with the best and most up-to-date information on arthritis treatments in an easy-to-read format that you could simply thumb through. We have included the best-of-the-best of many different healing systems — ranging from standard Western medicine (including medications and surgery), to Eastern healing systems (including Ayurvedic and Traditional Chinese methods), to alternative therapies (including homeopathy, herbs, and such far-out approaches as bee venom therapy). If you like, you can read this book straight through from cover-to-cover, but it's not absolutely necessary. We do suggest that you read the first chapter as an introduction, and then zero in on the description of your particular kind of arthritis, found in Chapter 2, 3, or 4. After that, feel free to flip through the book and read whatever catches your fancy.

Because arthritis impacts your life in so many different ways, we have chapters that address the many complex issues that you may face, including the technical aspects of arthritis (tests, medicines, and surgeries), the practical aspects (diet, exercise, and day-to-day living), and the emotional aspects (depression and anger). We also give tips on how to assemble your health-care treatment team, how to talk to your doctor, and what to do about chronic pain.

Our Assumptions about You

In writing this book, we made certain educated guesses about you, the reader, so that we could figure out what might be most interesting and useful to you and write our book accordingly. We've assumed that

- You either have arthritis yourself or you're close to someone who has it.
- You're interested in learning about arthritis and its treatments.
- You want to do something to ease arthritis pain and/or other symptoms.
- You want to play an active part in managing the disease, rather than just going along with whatever the doctor tells you.
- You're interested in finding out about some alternative ways to treat arthritis.
- You'd like to find out how to handle the emotional issues that go hand-in-hand with the disease.

How This Book Is Organized

The organization of *Arthritis for Dummies* is meant to correspond with the way that you may experience arthritis in your daily life. When you first realize that you have arthritis, you probably want to know what it is, what the common symptoms are, and what you might expect as the disease progresses. Next, you'll visit your doctor for tests. Medicines may be prescribed, pain management strategies discussed, and surgery (if applicable) may be mentioned.

But once you've made it through all that, you'll go back to living your life. Suddenly, the everyday things that you used to take for granted will become important parts of your arthritis management — like diet, exercise, and the way that you use your joints. Stress and depression may be new and confounding problems, and getting through the day may be a tougher prospect, both physically and mentally, than it was before.

Eventually, you may start wondering about alternative healing methods, and have an urge to explore them. And you may become curious about certain myths that you've heard repeated about super foods to help ease arthritis symptoms and cutting-edge medical treatments that are on the horizon. This book will answer all of your questions, in the order that they've arisen for many people.

Part I: What Type of Arthritis Do You Have?

These four chapters give an overview of arthritis in its many forms — the symptoms, disease processes, causes, and most likely victims. Chapter 1 discusses arthritis in general, Chapter 2 tackles osteoarthritis (the type of arthritis that most people get), Chapter 3 explains rheumatoid arthritis (another fairly common kind of arthritis), and Chapter 4 discusses the other forms the disease may take. We also explain what doctors do for each type of arthritis and what you can do for yourself.

Part II: Tests and Treatments: What to Expect from Your Doctor

Chapters 5 through 9 walk you through the maze of medical treatments, beginning with a trip to the doctor's office. We explain how doctors diagnose the many forms of arthritis and discuss the high-tech and low-tech tests that they may use. Equally important, we show you how to work with your doctor to make the treatment decisions. Chapter 7 outlines the medicines that may be prescribed and the surgeries that may be applicable. Finally, strategies that you can use at home for managing pain are thoroughly explained.

Part III: The Arthritis Lifestyle Strategy

Many of the keys to arthritis management lie in the little things that you do every day, such as what you eat, the kind and amount of exercise you get, and how you use your joints. In this part, we tell you how to fight arthritis pain through diet and supplements; how to keep your joints in shape through exercise; how to protect your joints by walking, sitting, and moving correctly; and how to deal effectively with depression and anger. Plus, we provide loads of tips on how to make day-to-day living with arthritis easier.

Part IV: Is Alternative Medicine for You?

Alternative medicine has become incredibly popular in the past 20 years, and scientific studies are beginning to show that many of these methods have merit. In this part, we discuss the most popular alternative therapies for arthritis, including massage, herbs, homeopathy, acupuncture, reflexology, traditional Chinese medicine, Ayurvedic healing, and others. We also give you tips on finding a reputable alternative practitioner and identifying false claims.

Part V: The Part of Tens

In this part, we concentrate some of the key information on managing your arthritis into four lists, each containing ten "information bites." We include ten arthritis myths, ten tips for management and prevention of arthritis, ten super foods that can help you fight arthritis, and ten crackerjack new treatments that you may not have heard about yet.

Part VI: Appendixes

Appendix A contains a glossary of arthritis terms to help keep you straight as you wend your way through the information in this book. Appendix B lists lots of interesting organizations that may help you find the treatment you seek. We give detailed information on the foundations associated with most kinds of arthritis or arthritis-related conditions, as well as major medical associations. We list the certifying boards or associations for each alternative therapy we discuss, so you can request practitioner referrals or more information. Information on support groups, mail order catalogues featuring assistive devices, books, and videotapes are all included in Appendix B.

Icons Used in This Book

The icons tell you what you must know, what you should know, and what you may find interesting but can live without.

When you see this icon, it means the information is essential and you should be aware of it.

This icon marks important information that can save you time and energy.

This icon marks whenever we tell a story about patients.

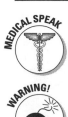

The Medical Speak icon marks a more in-depth, medical passage.

The Warning icon cautions you against potential problems.

This icon denotes paragraphs that define terms.

Where to Go from Here

Someone once said, "Knowledge is power." You have the power to take charge of your arthritis; all you have to do is educate yourself and apply what you learn. This book is a good place to start, but you'll have to commit and re-commit yourself to maintaining your health on a daily basis. Remember, it's the little things that you do every day that count. As you embark on your journey, we wish you luck, strength, and many active, pain-free years!

Part I

What Type of Arthritis Do You Have?

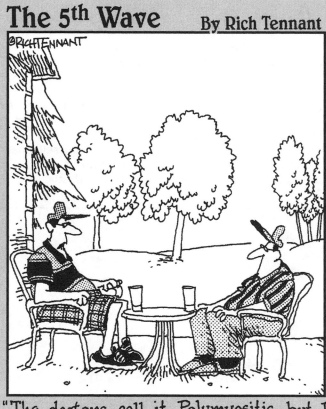

The 5th Wave   By Rich Tennant

"The doctors call it Polymyositis, but I call it 'Military Arthritis' because it comes with a lot of fatigue."

In this part . . .

Arthritis can really put a damper on your life . . . if you let it. But the good news is that most forms of arthritis and the pain they cause can be managed (if not completely done away with) through medical techniques and lifestyle changes.

Part I gives you an overview of arthritis in its many forms; the symptoms, diseases, processes, causes, and most likely victims. You also learn what doctors can do for each type of arthritis and what you can do for yourself. Special attention is given to the most common forms of this disease: osteoarthritis and rheumatoid arthritis.

Chapter 1

What Is Arthritis?

*O*uch! There it goes again! That grinding pain in your hip; those aching knees that make walking from the kitchen to the bedroom a chore; the stiff and swollen fingers that won't allow you to twist the lid off a sticky jar or even sew on a button. Arthritis seems to get to everybody sooner or later, slowing us down, forcing us to give up some of our favorite activities, and just generally being a pain in the neck (sometimes literally!). In more advanced cases, it can seriously compromise quality of life as sufferers surrender their independence, mobility, and sense of usefulness while being relentlessly worn down by pain.

The good news is that you can manage your arthritis, if not cure it, with a combination of medical care, simple lifestyle changes, and good old common sense. You don't have to spend your life sitting at home in an easy chair, gritting your teeth from pain, or hobbling around the backyard with a cane. Although you may not be able to run a marathon or do back-flips like you did when you were 13, if you follow the program outlined here, you should be able to do the things you really want to do — such as take a brisk walk in the park, carry a sleeping child upstairs to bed, or swing a golf club with the best of them. Arthritis may affect a lot of people, but thanks to intensive research over the past several years, we now know a lot more about how to handle it.

Arthritis Is More than Aching Joints

So what exactly is arthritis, this disease that brings us so much misery and pain? Unfortunately, there isn't one easy answer to that question because arthritis involves a *group* of diseases, each with its own cause, set of symptoms, and treatments. What these diseases *do* have in common is the following:

- ✔ They affect some part of the joint — the cartilage, bones, synovial membrane, bursae, tendons, ligaments, or muscles.
- ✔ They cause pain and (possibly) loss of movement.
- ✔ They often bring about some kind of inflammation (the *itis* in arthritis).

As for the causes of these different kinds of arthritis, they run the gamut from inheriting an unlucky gene to physical trauma to getting bitten by the wrong mosquito.

The word *arthritis*, which literally means joint inflammation, is derived from the Greek words *arthros* (joint) and *itis* (inflammation), and its major symptom is joint pain. Although the same group of ailments is sometimes called *rheumatism*, it's usually referred to as *arthritis*, so that's what we call it in this book. According to The Arthritis Foundation, some 40 million Americans (that's one out of every seven people) are affected by arthritis, and nearly 60 million will be afflicted by the year 2020. That's a big chunk of the population.

Say hello to your joints

Before you can understand what's wrong with your joints, you need to understand what a joint is and how it works. Any place in the body where two bones meet is called a *joint*. Bones are living tissue — hard, porous structures with a blood supply and nerves — that constantly rebuild themselves. Bones protect our vital organs and provide the supporting framework for the body. Without bones, we would be nothing more than blobs of tissue — like tents without supporting poles!

Defining a joint is easy: it's just a place where two bones come together. Sometimes those bones actually fuse, such as the bones of the skull. But in the joints that can develop arthritis, the bones don't actually touch. As you can see in Figure 1-1, there's a small amount of space between the two bone ends. The space between the ends of the bones keeps them from grinding against each other and wearing each other down.

But bones are more than broomsticks that prop us up, leaving us rigid and awkward. The 200-plus bones that reside in our bodies are connected together in some 150 joints, giving us remarkable flexibility and range of motion. If you don't believe it, just watch a gymnast, ballet dancer, or figure skater execute a handspring, arabesque, or triple axel. But you don't have to be an athlete or contortionist to enjoy the benefits of joint flexibility. Just think about some of the things you do regularly — such as twisting around while you sit in the front seat of your car to grab something off the backseat floor. Now imagine how limiting it would be if you had fewer joints, or if they didn't move the way they do!

Other structures surrounding the joint, such as the muscles, tendons, and bursae — small sacs that cushion the tendons — support the joint and provide the power that makes the bones move. The joint capsule wraps itself around the joint and its special lining, the synovial membrane or *synovium* makes a slick, slippery liquid called the *synovial fluid*. This liquid fills that little space between the bone ends. Finally, the bone ends are capped by cartilage — a slick, tough, rubbery material that is eight times more slippery than ice and a better shock absorber than the tires and springs on your car! Together, these parts make up the joint, one of the most fascinating bits of machinery found in the body.

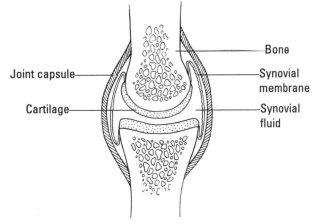

Figure 1-1:
Anatomy of
a normal
joint.

Cartilage: The human shock absorber

Cartilage is extremely important for the healthy functioning of a joint, especially if that joint bears weight, like your knee. Imagine for a moment that you're looking into the inner workings of your left knee as you walk down the street. When you shift your weight from your left leg to your right, the pressure on your left knee is released. The cartilage in your left knee then "drinks in" synovial fluid, in much the same way that a sponge soaks up liquid when immersed in water. When you take another step and transfer the weight back onto your left leg, much of the fluid squeezes out of the cartilage. This squeezing of joint fluid into and out of the cartilage helps it respond to the off-and-on pressure of walking without shattering under the strain.

Can you imagine the results if we didn't have this watery cushion within our joints? With the rough, porous surfaces of the bone ends pitted against each other, bones would grind each other down in no time. One thing is certain: nobody would be getting around too easily without joint fluid and cartilage.

Types of joints

To accommodate the bends, twists, and turns that we all perform without even thinking, the skeletal system is made up of different shapes and sizes of bones that connect to form different kinds of joints. The joints are categorized according to how much motion they allow:

- *Synarthroidal joints* allow no movement at all. You can find these in the skull, where the bones meet to form tough, fibrous joints called *sutures*. Because they don't move, arthritis doesn't affect them.

- *Amphiarthroidal joints,* such as those in the spine or the pelvis, allow limited movement. Generally, these joints aren't attacked by arthritic conditions as often as others. (A "slipped disc" is not arthritis.)

- *Synovial joints* allow a wide range of movement; most of our joints fall into this class. Synovial joints come in all kinds of interesting variations including those that glide, hinge, pivot, look like saddles, or have a ball-and-socket type structure. Because of the synovial joints, you can bend over and pick a flower, kick up your heels while swing dancing, reach for a glass on a high shelf, and turn around to see what's going on behind you. Unfortunately, these joints are also the ones most likely to be hit with arthritis, precisely because they do move!

Types of synovial joints

Because of their tendency to become arthritic, synovial joints are the ones that we discuss the most throughout this book. Synovial joints come in a wide variety of shapes and sizes to accommodate a wide variety of movements.

Gliding joints

A gliding joint contains two bones with somewhat flat surfaces that can slide over each other. The vertebrae in your spine are connected by gliding joints, allowing you to bend forward to touch your toes and backward to do a backbend (well, maybe!). See Figure 1-2 for an example of a gliding joint.

Hinge joints

You can find hinge joints in your elbows, knees, and fingers. These joints open and close like a door. But just like a door, hinge joints only go one way — you can't bend your knee up toward your face, only back toward your rear. See Figure 1-3 for an example of a hinge joint.

Some fun facts: Did you know . . .

✔ By the time a fetus is four months old, its joints and limbs are in working order and ready to move.

✔ A newborn baby has 350 bones, many of which fuse to form the 206 bones of the adult body.

✔ Cartilage is 65 percent to 80 percent water.

✔ When you run, the pressure on your knees can increase to ten times that of your body weight.

✔ There's not a single man-made substance that's more resilient, a better shock absorber, or lower in friction than cartilage.

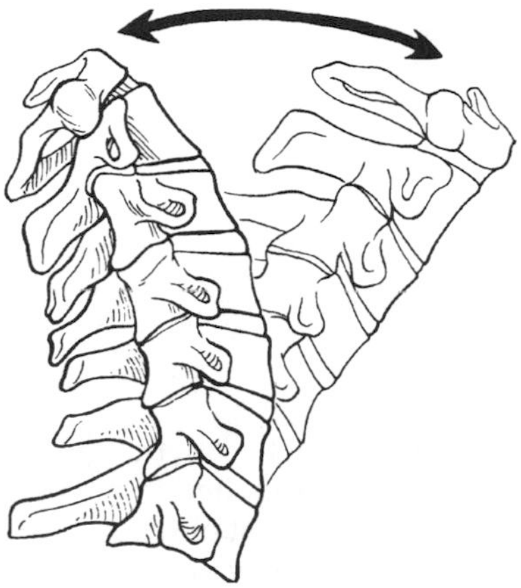

Figure 1-2:
A gliding joint. The gliding joint helps keep your vertebrae aligned when you bend and stretch.

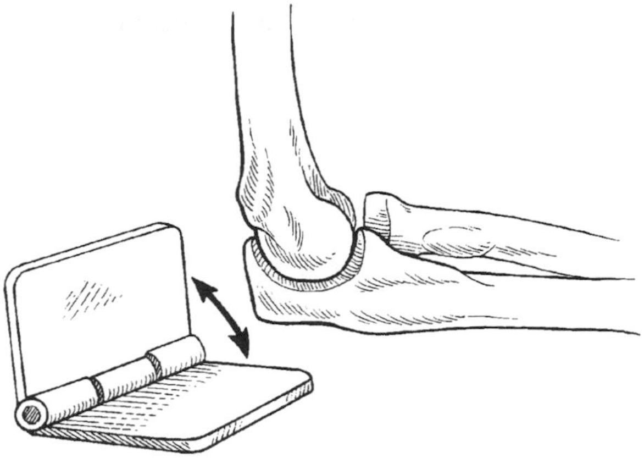

Figure 1-3:
A hinge joint. Hinge joints only bend one way.

Saddle joints

This joint got its name because it looks like a horse's back with a saddle resting on it. One bone is rounded (convex) and fits neatly into the other bone, which is concave. The saddle joint moves up and down and side to side, but it doesn't rotate. Your wrist and your thumb have this kind of joint. See Figure 1-4 for an example of a saddle joint.

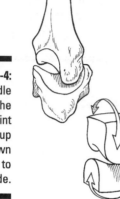

Figure 1-4:
A saddle joint. The saddle joint moves up and down and side to side.

Ball-and-socket joints

This is truly a freewheeling joint — it's ready for anything! Up, down, back, forth, or around in circles. The bone that's attached to a ball-and-socket joint can move in just about any direction. The end of one bone is round, like a ball, whereas the other bone has a neat little cave that the ball fits into. Your shoulders and hips have ball-and-socket joints. Being able to swim the backstroke is a perfect example of the kind of range of motion made possible by these joints. See Figure 1-5 for an example of a ball-and-socket joint.

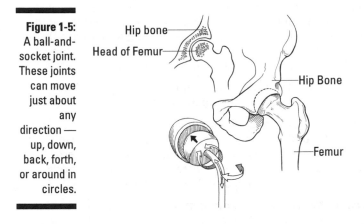

Hip bone

Head of Femur

Hip Bone

Femur

Arthritis and Arthritis-Related Conditions

Some organizations define arthritis as a group of more than 100 related diseases, ranging from bursitis to osteoarthritis. But in this book, we use the following classifications, which conform to those widely accepted by the medical community:

- ✔ true arthritis
- ✔ arthritis as a major player
- ✔ arthritis as a minor player
- ✔ arthritis as a companion condition

Here's a quick look at the various types of arthritis and arthritis-related diseases and their classifications. We'll discuss each disease in greater detail in Chapters 2, 3, and 4.

True arthritis

The following include conditions in which arthritis is the major part of the syndrome and the primary disease process:

- ✔ *Ankylosing spondylitis:* A chronic inflammation of the spine, this disease can cause the vertebrae to grow together, making the spine rigid. Although the cause is unknown, heredity is a factor.

- ✔ *Gout:* This "regal" form of arthritis is caused by the build-up of a substance called uric acid, which forms sharp crystals that are deposited in the joint. These needle-like crystals cause severe pain and are most commonly found in the "bunion" joint of the big toe, the knees, and the wrists. Genetic factors, diet, or certain drugs may cause gout.

- ✔ *Infectious arthritis:* Bacteria, viruses, or fungi that enter the body can settle in the joints, causing fever, inflammation, and loss of joint function.

- ✔ *Juvenile arthritis:* This is a catch-all term for the different kinds of arthritis that strike children under the age of 16, the most common of which is *juvenile rheumatoid arthritis* (JRA). Pain or swelling in the shoulders, elbows, knees, ankles or toes, chills, a reappearing fever, and sometimes a body rash are the typical symptoms of JRA. The cause is unknown.

- ✔ *Osteoarthritis:* In this, the most common type of arthritis, the cartilage breaks down, exposing bone ends and allowing them to rub together. The result can be pain, stiffness, loss of movement, and sometimes swelling. Osteoarthritis is most often found in the weight-bearing joints, such as the hips, knees, ankles, and spine, but it can also affect the fingers. It may be the result of trauma, metabolic conditions, obesity, heredity, or other factors.

- ✔ *Pseudogout:* Like gout, pseudogout is caused by the deposition of crystals into the joint, but instead of uric acid crystals, they're made from calcium. Pain, swelling, and sometimes the destruction of cartilage can result.

- ✔ *Psoriatic Arthritis:* This form of arthritis occurs in people who have the inherited skin condition called *psoriasis*, which causes scaly, red, rough patches on the neck, elbows, and knees, as well as the pitting of the nails. Often settling in the joints of the fingers and toes, psoriatic arthritis can cause the digits to swell up like little sausages.

- ✔ *Rheumatoid arthritis:* In this, the second-most common form of arthritis, the immune system turns against the body, causing inflammation and swelling that begins in the joint lining and spreads to the cartilage and the bone. It often affects the same joint on both sides of the body (for example, both wrists).

Arthritis as a major player

In the following conditions, arthritis is present and is usually a major part of the syndrome, but is *not* the primary disease process:

- ✔ *Lyme disease:* Caused by a certain type of bacteria transmitted to humans via a tick bite, Lyme disease brings about fever, a distinctive red skin lesion in the shape of a bull's-eye, problems with the nerves and/or heart, and arthritis. Antibiotics are the treatment of choice for this disease.

✔ *Reiter's syndrome:* An inflammation of the joints, Reiter's strikes along with or shortly after the onset of a sexually-transmitted or intestinal infection. The classic trio of Reiter's problems are arthritis, conjunctivitis (inflammation of the eyelid's lining), and urethritis (inflammation of the urethra).

✔ *Scleroderma:* The word *scleroderma* means *hard skin*. When tiny capillaries and blood vessels become inflamed and the body responds by overproducing collagen, the skin, blood, internal organs, and joints can suffer. The joint stiffness in scleroderma is actually due to the hardening of the skin. An autoimmune disease, scleroderma usually attacks adults rather than children.

✔ *Systemic lupus erythematosus:* This is yet another disease caused by an immune system gone wrong. In lupus the body attacks its own connective tissue causing inflammation, joint pain, stiffness, permanent damage to the joints, and exhaustion. The disease usually makes itself known during a woman's childbearing years.

Arthritis as a minor player

In these conditions, arthritis may appear, but it is a minor part of the syndrome.

✔ *Bursitis and Tendonitis:* Caused by overusing or injuring a joint, bursitis is the inflammation of the fibrous sac that cushions the tendons. Tendonitis is the irritation of the tendons, which attach the muscles to the bones.

✔ *Paget's disease:* With Paget's disease, the breakdown and rebuilding of bone speeds up. The resulting bone is larger but also softer and weaker, making it more likely to fracture. These weakened and deformed bones cause arthritis to develop in their respective joints, which typically include those of the hip, skull, spine, knee, and ankle. The cause is unknown.

✔ *Polymyalgia Rheumatica:* Seemingly overnight, severe stiffness may strike in the hips, shoulders, and neck, making it difficult even to get out of bed. Headaches, scalp tenderness, hearing problems, jaw pain, difficulty swallowing, and coughing are all symptoms of this disease of unknown origin.

✔ *Raynaud's disease and Raynaud's phenomenon:* Prompted by arterial spasm, Raynaud's can turn the fingers, toes, and other areas blue or red and cause tingling, numbness, burning, and/or a "pins and needles" sensation. If it happens on its own, it's called Raynaud's disease. If it strikes in conjunction with or appears to be caused by scleroderma, rheumatic arthritis, or other disorders, it's called Raynaud's phenomenon.

> ✔ *Sjogren's syndrome:* Another autoimmune disease, Sjogren's syndrome brings about inflammation of the tear glands and saliva glands, causing dryness of the eyes and mouth, hazy vision, cracks at the corners of the mouth, as well as problems chewing and swallowing. Inflammation of the brain, nerves, thyroid, lungs, liver, kidneys, and, of course, the joints may also be present.

Arthritis as a companion condition

In these conditions, arthritis may be present, but it constitutes another separate disease process.

> ✔ *Carpal Tunnel Syndrome:* This syndrome results when pressure on a nerve in the wrist makes the fingers tingle and feel numb. This syndrome is usually caused by overuse of the wrist. Permanent muscle and nerve damage can occur if carpal tunnel isn't treated.
>
> ✔ *Fibromyalgia:* This is an inflammation of the connective tissue of the muscles, tendons and bones. Fibromyalgia can make you "hurt all over," particularly in certain tender points in the neck, upper back, elbows, and knees. Those with fibromyalgia can suffer from disturbed sleep, fatigue, stiffness, and depression. The cause is unknown. Physical or mental stress, fatigue, or infections may trigger this disease.
>
> ✔ *Myositis:* This disease causes inflammation of the muscles, which can take one of two forms: *polymyositis* — an inflammation of the muscle that causes muscle weakening and breakdown as well as pain, and *dermatomyositis* — polymyositis plus rashes that can lead to skin scarring and changes in pigmentation.

Is It Really Arthritis? Signs and Symptoms

With all the different kinds of arthritis, how do you know if you have one of them? Arthritis can strike anyone at any time, and many times it's difficult to tell whether the pain is serious enough to warrant medical attention. Almost everyone has had an ache or pain at some time or has overextended himself or herself physically, but it's important to know what is minor and temporary, and what may be serious and long term. Learning what to watch for can make a difference in your treatment and physical comfort. Typical warning signs of arthritis are

> ✔ **Joint pain:** This not only includes steady, ever-present pain, but also off-again-on-again pain, pain that occurs only when you're moving or only when you're sitting still. In fact, if your joints hurt in *any* way for more than two weeks, you should see your doctor.

✔ **Stiffness or difficulty in moving a joint:** If you have trouble getting out of bed, unscrewing a jar lid, climbing the stairs, or doing anything else that involves moving your joints, consider it a red flag. Although difficulty moving a joint is most often the result of a muscular condition, it could be a sign of arthritis.

✔ **Swelling:** If the skin around a joint is red, puffed up, hot, throbbing, or painful to the touch, you're experiencing joint inflammation. Don't wait. See your doctor.

The warning signs may come in triplicate (pain plus stiffness plus swelling), two together, or one all alone. Or, as you find out in Chapters 3 and 4, there may be other early signs such as malaise or muscle pain. But if you experience *any* of these or other symptoms in or around a joint for longer than two weeks, you should see your doctor.

What Causes Arthritis?

Just as there are many different kinds of arthritis, there are many different causes — and some of them are still unknown. But in general, scientists have found that certain factors can contribute to the development of joint problems:

✔ **Heredity:** Your parents gave you your beautiful eyes, strong jaw-line, exceptional math ability and, possibly, a tendency to develop rheumatoid arthritis. Scientists have discovered that the genetic marker HLA-DR4 is linked to rheumatoid arthritis, so if you happen to have this gene, you're more likely to develop the disease. Ankylosing spondylitis is linked to the genetic marker HLA-B27, and although having this gene doesn't mean that you absolutely will get this form of arthritis, you can if conditions are right.

✔ **Age:** It's just a fact of life that the older you get, the more likely you are to develop arthritis, especially osteoarthritis. Like the tires on your car, cartilage can wear down over time, becoming thin, cracked, or even wearing through. Bones may also break down with age, bringing on joint pain and dysfunction.

✔ **Overuse of a joint:** What do ballerinas, baseball pitchers, and tennis players all have in common? A great chance that they'll develop arthritis due to the tremendous repetitive strain they put on their joints. The dancers, who go from flat foot to "pointe" hundreds of times during a practice session, eventually end up with painful arthritic ankles. Baseball pitchers, throwing fastballs at speeds of more than 100 mph, regularly develop arthritis of the shoulder and/or elbow. And you don't need to be a tennis pro to develop tennis elbow, a form of tendonitis that has sidelined many a player.

✔ **Injury:** Sustaining injury to a joint (from a household mishap, a car accident, playing sports, or doing anything else) increases the odds that you could develop arthritis in that joint in the future. Football players are well-known victims of arthritis of the knee, and it's certainly not surprising. They often fall smack on their knees or other joints when they are tackled — then have a ton of "football flesh" crash down on top of them. What's most amazing is that they sometimes walk away uninjured.

✔ **Infection:** Some forms of arthritis are the result of bacteria, viruses, or fungi that can either cause the disease or trigger it in susceptible people. Lyme disease comes from bacteria transmitted by the bite of a tick. Rheumatoid arthritis may come from a virus that triggers it in people with a certain genetic marker. Infectious arthritis can arise following surgery, trauma, a needle inserted into the joint, bone infection, or an infection that's traveled from another area of the body.

✔ **Tumor Necrosis Factor (TNF):** TNF is a substance the body produces that causes inflammation and may play a part in initiating or maintaining rheumatoid arthritis. Although scientists are unsure exactly what triggers rheumatoid arthritis, they have found that drugs that counteract the effects of TNF, called TNF antagonists, are often helpful in managing the symptoms of this disease.

Who Gets Arthritis?

Statistically speaking, the typical arthritis victim (if there were such a thing) would be a middle-class Caucasian woman between the ages of 65 and 74 who has a high school education, is overweight, is a city-dweller in the southern United States, and has osteoarthritis. The least likely to develop arthritis would be a Native American male under the age of 16 who lives in the Northeast and has a family income of more than $50,000.

But arthritis isn't all that picky, and doesn't worry too much about statistics. It strikes both young and old, male and female, rich and poor, and doesn't seem to care where you live. Arthritis, in one form or another, can affect just about anybody.

However, arthritis does seem to hit women particularly hard. Nearly two-thirds of those who get the disease are women — an estimated 26 million Americans. Some facts about women and arthritis:

✔ Arthritis affects 8.6 percent of women age 15-44, 33.5 percent of women age 45-64 and 55.8 percent of women over the age of 65.

✔ Arthritis limits the daily activities of an estimated 4.6 million women.

> ✔ Some 15.3 million women are currently affected by osteoarthritis, a disease that strikes women nearly three times more often than men.
>
> ✔ Seventy-one percent of rheumatoid arthritis patients are women, about 1.5 million.
>
> ✔ Nearly 86 percent of juvenile rheumatoid arthritis cases are found in girls.

Additionally, arthritis affects some 4 million African Americans. African Americans rank arthritis as the third most prevalent health condition affecting them, topped only by high blood pressure and chronic sinus problems. It was placed ahead of heart disease, diabetes, and asthma, among others. They are also more likely than other racial groups to experience limited activities due to arthritis.

African American women are at particular risk for arthritis. There's a higher rate of arthritis reported among African American women after age 35 than in Caucasian women, and young African American women are three times more likely to develop lupus than their Caucasian counterparts.

Arthritis facts

✔ Forty million Americans currently suffer from arthritis, or 1 in 6 of us. This figure is expected to rise to nearly 60 million (1 in 5) by 2020.

✔ Osteoarthritis leads the pack in prevalence, affecting nearly 21 million Americans, most of whom develop the disease after the age of 45.

✔ Women are nearly twice as likely as men to suffer from arthritis.

✔ Rheumatoid arthritis (RA) and gout are tied for third, at 2.1 million Americans. But RA strikes mostly women, while gout tends to favor men.

✔ Gout is twice as likely to strike African-American men as Caucasian men, possibly because African-American men are more likely to use medicines to lower blood pressure. These drugs increase production of uric acid, which can crystallize and settle painfully in joints.

✔ Those who live in the city are three times more likely to develop arthritis than those who live in rural areas.

✔ The number of children under the age of 17 who have arthritis is an astonishing 285,000, including 50,000 who have juvenile rheumatoid arthritis (JRA).

✔ The lower your income, the more likely you are to develop arthritis. According to the Arthritis Foundation, 20.3 percent of those with an annual income of less than $10,000 had arthritis, as opposed to 13.4 percent of those who made $50,000 or more.

Famous people who suffer from arthritis

Does the idea of having arthritis make you feel like you may as well just give up? Well, that's what a lot of people could have done, but didn't. Here are some examples of what some people have done with their lives while coping with arthritis:

- **Lucille Ball** was diagnosed with rheumatoid arthritis at the age of 17, but she went on to live a long and healthy life, enjoying a top-notch career in movies and television.

- The famous French artist **Pierre-Auguste Renoir** also developed RA in his late 50's, but painted nearly 6,000 pictures during his lifetime, many of them great masterpieces.

- Actress **Mary McDonough**, best known for her role as Erin on the TV show *The Waltons*, has lupus yet is a wife and mother and continues a successful career as an actress and spokesperson for the Lupus Foundation of America.

- **Dr. Christian Barnard** developed rheumatoid arthritis as a youngster but went on to perform the world's first human heart transplant in 1967.

- **Billie Jean King** has osteoarthritis of the knees, probably the result of a car accident when she was 18 years old. Yet she won the Wimbledon singles title for the sixth time when she was in her early thirties and successfully took on Bobby Riggs in the "Battle of the Sexes" tennis tournament.

- **Norman Cousins**, editor of the *Saturday Review*, developed ankylosing spondylitis in 1964. As part of his then unheard of treatment, he watched Three Stooges, the Marx Brothers, and *Candid Camera* to make himself laugh and keep his spirits up. The book he later penned, called *Anatomy of an Illness,* became a bestseller, and he lived a long and productive life.

- **Rosalind Russell,** star of the silver screen, suffered from severe RA and did much to garner support for the advancement of research into this disease.

- **Wayne Gretsky**, possibly the greatest hockey player of all time, suffers from early signs of osteoarthritis.

- **Grandma Moses** had arthritis in her hands at age 76 when she began painting the folksy, whimsical scenes of American life that made her famous. Despite her condition, she created hundreds of paintings, many of which hang today in major museums all over the world.

You're Not Alone: Accepting Your Diagnosis

The good news is that arthritis can be managed in many cases. It may take some time and effort to find the right treatment(s) for your particular version of the disease, but there are answers. Although your doctor may recommend medication to help relieve the pain, there are also many things you can do yourself to keep the pain at bay and, perhaps, prevent further damage and help your joints heal. There are several treatment strategies, including foods that help you heal, exercises that can help lubricate your joints, joint protection techniques, alternative treatments, and surgery. By the time you finish reading this book, you and your health care team should be able to put together an "Arthritis Lifestyle Plan" tailored specifically to your needs — one that can help put you on the road to joint health for the rest of your life.

Chapter 2

Osteoarthritis: The Most Common Form

*W*hether it's called degenerative arthritis, degenerative joint disease, or osteoarthritis, simply put, osteoarthritis is the painful result of cartilage breakdown. When the tough, rubbery substance that cushions bone ends no longer does its job, the bone ends can't slide across each other easily within the joint. That's when pain and stiffness can settle into a joint. Suddenly, your knee aches, your hip burns, a finger joint swells and throbs, or your shoulder stiffens up. You can't bend and flex the painful joint like you used to; its range of movement is limited. Most of all, it just plain hurts!

But what happened to mess up your cartilage in the first place? To understand what went wrong, here's a look at how things work in healthy cartilage.

It's the Cartilage That Does It

Healthy cartilage is absolutely essential for joints to function properly and painlessly. Slick as a polished marble and tough as galvanized rubber, cartilage protects the ends of your bones from wearing each other away where they meet inside a joint. It also provides a smooth, slick surface so bone ends can glide easily across each other. And, cartilage is an excellent shock absorber, cushioning the bones and soaking up the impact created by movement and physical stresses. Without intact cartilage, bones grind away at each other and bear the brunt of the impact of movement. Eventually, the joint itself can be damaged or even destroyed.

Four elements help cartilage do its all-important job: water, collagen, proteoglycans, and chondrocytes, as follows:

- ✔ **Water:** Sixty-five to 80 percent of cartilage is water — a crucial substance that lubricates the joints, cushions bones, and absorbs shock.

- ✔ **Collagen:** Elasticity and a superb capability to absorb shock make collagen an integral part of healthy cartilage. A connective tissue that helps hold bones, muscles, and other bodily structures together; collagen is the mesh-like framework that provides a home for the proteoglycans.

- ✔ **Proteoglycans:** Large, oblong-shaped molecules that are covered with centipede-like "arms" that weave themselves securely into the collagen mesh and soak up water like a sponge. Then, when pressured, they release water. Thanks in part to the proteoglycans, cartilage can mold itself to the shape of the joint and respond to the ever-changing amount of pressure within the joint capsule.

- ✔ **Chondrocytes:** These cells follow the principle "out with the old and in with the new" as they break down and get rid of old proteoglycan and collagen molecules, forming new ones to take their place.

Water, collagen, proteoglycans, and chondrocytes all work together to keep your joints moving like well-oiled machinery. When the pressure is released from a joint, say your knee when you lift your leg to take a step, water rushes into the cartilage, nourishing, bathing, and plumping it up. The water-loving proteoglycans, woven securely into the collagen web, soak up water and hold on to it until pressure is applied to the joint (that is, you take another step). Then the water and wastes rush out of the cartilage. But as soon as the pressure is off, the proteoglycans thirstily soak up the water again. The resilient collagen stretches and shrinks to accommodate joint pressure and water content, so your cartilage can bounce back after being flattened out.

But if your cartilage loses its ability to attract and hold water, it becomes thin, dry, cracked, and unable to provide a slippery surface. No longer plump and resilient, it makes a poor shock absorber and cushion for the bones, which particularly affects the weight-bearing joints.

You can visualize the action of the cartilage by thinking of two cans of soup facing each other end-to-end with an almost-filled water balloon in between them. As you press the soup cans together, the water balloon changes shape to accommodate the pressure, but never lets the cans actually touch. When you release the pressure, the water balloon (like your cartilage) resumes its old shape. See Figure 2-1 for a diagram of a healthy joint and Figure 2-2 for a picture of an unhealthy joint.

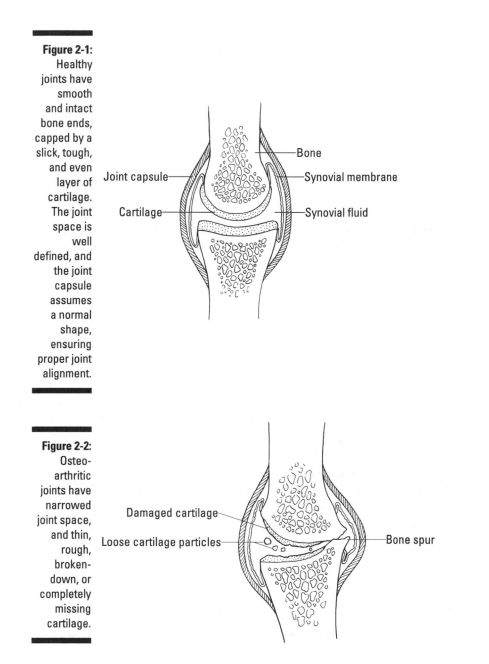

Figure 2-1:
Healthy joints have smooth and intact bone ends, capped by a slick, tough, and even layer of cartilage. The joint space is well defined, and the joint capsule assumes a normal shape, ensuring proper joint alignment.

Bone

Joint capsule

Synovial membrane

Cartilage

Synovial fluid

Figure 2-2:
Osteo-arthritic joints have narrowed joint space, and thin, rough, broken-down, or completely missing cartilage.

Damaged cartilage

Loose cartilage particles

Bone spur

Warning Signs and Symptoms of Osteoarthritis

Don't assume that you have osteoarthritis just because you have one or more of the following symptoms. Get a thorough examination and diagnosis from a qualified physician. Figure 2-3 shows you the most common sites affected by osteoarthritis.

How do you know if the joint pain you're suffering from is due to osteoarthritis? Most of those with the disease have at least one of the following symptoms:

- ✔ **Joint pain:** Most people experience joint pain as a deep-seated ache radiating from the inner core of the joint. It's a distinctly different feeling than a muscular ache and may come and go according to changes in the weather. ("I can feel it in my bones that it's going to rain.") The pain typically increases as the joint is used and eases off with joint rest. As the disease worsens, though, the pain can become fairly steady. If joint pain occurs during the night, poor sleep and next-day fatigue may be two unpleasant side effects.

- ✔ **Stiffness and loss of movement:** Stiff joints, limited range of motion and, in later stages, joints that freeze into a bent position are all signs of osteoarthritis.

- ✔ **Tenderness, warmth, and swelling around the joint:** Although swelling is not usually a big problem with osteoarthritis, some joints do swell in response to cartilage damage and irritation, especially if they've been overused. The finger joints and the knees are most often affected.

- ✔ **"Cracking" joints:** If you hear popping or crunching sounds when you move a joint, you may have osteoarthritis. These cracking sounds (doctors call them *crepitus*) can be created by roughened cartilage.

- ✔ **Bony growths on the fingers:** Bony lumps, either at the ends of the fingers (called *Heberden's nodes*) or on the middle joint of the fingers (called *Bouchard's nodes*) are signs of osteoarthritis. These types of bony growths may be hereditary.

Some people really can feel it in their joints when it's going to rain. That's because as the barometric pressure falls, the lining of an arthritic joint can become inflamed, causing pain and the release of excess fluid (swelling).

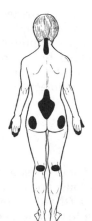

Figure 2-3:
The neck, lower back, knees, hips, ends of the fingers, and the thumbs are the most common sites affected by osteo-arthritis.

What Causes Cartilage Breakdown?

Sometimes, we really don't know why the cartilage disintegrates. In that case, we designate the problem as *primary osteoarthritis*, or osteoarthritis of unknown cause. Other times we know that the osteoarthritis has been triggered by another problem, in which case we call it *secondary osteoarthritis*.

Primary osteoarthritis

The ultimate cause of primary osteoarthritis remains a mystery. Although scientists aren't sure why, the collagen mesh of the cartilage becomes scrambled; it weakens and can't hold its structure. The proteoglycans, once so cozily intertwined in the collagen mesh, suddenly find themselves evicted from their secure homes. As they float off into the joint fluid, they take their water-retaining abilities with them. The cartilage is left high and dry; it thins and may even crack. At the same time, the newly-freed proteoglycans draw excess fluid into the joint capsule, causing swelling. (Unfortunately, this fluid can't get back into the cartilage, where it's desperately needed. It's something like dying of thirst in the middle of the ocean.)

Although no one is absolutely certain what causes primary osteoarthritis, here are a few theories:

⮕ **The chondrocytes become too efficient at breaking down the collagen and proteoglycan molecules:** In healthy cartilage, the amount of breaking down enzymes is equal to the amount of building up enzymes. An over-abundance of destructive enzymes leads to weakened collagen and a lack of proteoglycans.

✔ **The chondrocytes go wild and start making too many proteoglycan and collagen molecules:** The opposite of the previous condition, these chondrocytes are too good at making new cartilage components. The excess proteoglycan and collagen molecules, in turn, pull extra fluid into the joint, flooding it and washing away most of the chondrocytes. The cartilage, then, is left bereft of cartilage-producing molecules.

Secondary osteoarthritis

Although the origins of primary osteoarthritis remain murky, experts are quite sure what causes secondary osteoarthritis: various types of trauma to the joints. That includes sudden, high-velocity trauma (the kind you'd experience in a car accident) as well as little insults to your joints that occur time and again, like repeated poor posture or running on a concrete surface every day for years. The causes of secondary osteoarthritis can be further broken down as follows:

✔ **Joint injury:** Weekend warriors beware! Once a joint has been injured, be it through a sports mishap, car accident, household slippage, or anything else, it is much more likely to develop osteoarthritis.

✔ **Repetitive motion injury:** Joints that are stressed over and over again in the same way (for example, a ballerina's ankles, a football player's knees, or a data processor's wrists) are more likely to experience a cartilage breakdown than joints subjected to normal use.

✔ **Damage to the bone end:** Usually due to trauma or continual stress, a bone may chip or sustain small fractures. In the body's zeal to repair the damage, it may cause an overgrowth of bone in the injured area. The result is a bone end that's bumpy, not smooth, and joint problems can ensue.

✔ **Bone disease:** A bone disease, such as Paget's disease, weakens the bone structure, making it more likely to fracture and develop bony overgrowth.

✔ **Carrying too much body weight:** The heavier you are, the more stress your knees, hips, and ankles must bear. Osteoarthritis of the knee has been clearly linked to excess body weight. That's not surprising considering that every time you take a step the stress on your knee is roughly equivalent to three times your body weight. Increase that figure to 10 when you run!

The repair problem

To make matters worse, once your cartilage is damaged, your body can compound the problem by the way it repairs itself. Like injured bone, injured cartilage can overdo the repair process, piling too much new cartilage into a crack or tear. The result is a lumpy, bumpy surface that doesn't glide smoothly against the cartilage on the opposing bone end. On the other hand, sometimes the cartilage doesn't repair itself at all, and remains in its damaged state — cracked, pitted, frayed, and even worn-through. Pieces of loose cartilage and/or bone may break off and float freely through the joint fluid. The bone-ends, no longer well cushioned, start to rub against each other and can develop bony spurs (osteophytes) that further interfere with smooth joint movement. The joint space narrows and the entire shape of the joint can change. All this from a little damaged cartilage!

You may hear your doctor use a few technical terms, such as: *eburnation,* which is increased and abnormal bone density; *subchondral bone,* which is the bone right below the cartilage; or *subchondral cyst,* which is an abnormal pocket of fluid in the bone beneath the cartilage.

Who Gets It? Risk factors

Not everybody gets osteoarthritis. Some people actually sail into their golden years with joints unaffected by pain, stiffness, or other symptoms, while others are hobbling around by the time they're 35. So how come one person gets osteoarthritis while another gets away scot-free? And how can you tell if you happen to be particularly susceptible to it?

Your chances of developing osteoarthritis are increased if:

- ✔ **You're past age 45:** Cartilage and other joint structures, like most bodily tissues, tend to degrade and become weaker over time. After decades of use, they start to wear out. Luckily, research has shown that osteoarthritis is not inevitable as we age. The odds just go up.

- ✔ **You've had a joint injury:** If you've been in a car accident, have played rough-and-tumble sports, or have injured any of your joints in any way, you will be more likely to develop osteoarthritis in the joints that were affected by those activities.

- ✔ **Your joints have been repeatedly stressed:** Ballet dancers, assembly line workers, baseball pitchers, grocery checkers, and anyone else who overuses and stresses a joint or joints can suffer from cartilage breakdown in those joints.

- ✔ **You're a woman:** Women are three times more likely than men to develop osteoarthritis. This may be due to smaller joint structures or some link to estrogen; nothing has yet been proven.

- ✔ **Your parents had it:** There appears to be a genetic component to osteoarthritis; in fact, one study concluded that genes were responsible for 50 percent of hip osteoarthritis. Osteoarthritis in the hands is also believed to be at least partially due to genetics. An inherited tendency toward defective cartilage or poorly structured joints can certainly put you on the road to osteoarthritis, although it doesn't necessarily mean that you'll eventually develop it.

✔ **You're overweight:** Excess weight puts a great deal of strain on the weight-bearing joints — the hips, knees, and ankles. For every ten pounds of excess weight you carry, you increase the force exerted on these joints anywhere from three to ten times, depending upon the type of activity. Researchers have found a definite link between being overweight and osteoarthritis, especially involving the knee joint.

Is It Really Osteoarthritis? The Diagnosis

Nearly 50 percent of those suffering from osteoarthritis don't know what kind of arthritis they have and therefore can't make good decisions about their treatment.

Say your knee hurts. The first time that you visit your doctor complaining of the pain, he will put you through the standard round of interviews, examinations, and tests. He'll review your medical history, and make a detailed list of the injuries you have sustained, especially to your knees. He may palpate your knee to see if it's painful to the touch, carefully bend your knee and straighten it several times (it may hurt a little and seem stiff), and listen for cracking or popping in the joint. Then, your doctor may send you to the lab to get some blood drawn to rule out other forms of arthritis. At this point, all your doctor has to go on is a history of knee injuries, some pain and stiffness upon movement, and a little cracking in the joint. It certainly may sound like osteoarthritis, but it may not yet be a sure thing.

The next step would be to order an X ray of your knee to see if one or more of the following signs are present:

✔ Cartilage degradation

✔ Cartilage overgrowth

✔ Narrowing of the joint space

✔ Bone spurs

✔ Bits of cartilage or bone floating in the joint fluid

✔ Joint deformity

Treating Osteoarthritis

After a diagnosis of osteoarthritis is confirmed, you and your doctor can begin to devise a treatment program — confident that you are headed in the right direction. Although the symptoms may not disappear completely, there is a good chance that with proper treatment your pain will diminish significantly and joint degradation can be kept to a minimum.

A good treatment plan for osteoarthritis should include the following elements to help you manage pain and discomfort on a daily basis.

Medication

Both prescription and over-the-counter remedies are commonly used to relieve osteoarthritis pain. Whether prescription or nonprescription, the drugs usually fall into one or two categories:

✔ *Acetaminophen:* (for example — Tylenol, Liquiprin, or Datril) These relieve pain but don't reduce swelling.

✔ *Nonsteroidal anti-inflammatories or NSAIDs:* (for example, aspirin, Advil, Aleve, or Motrin) These relieve pain and do reduce swelling, as well as lessen fever.

If your joints are swollen, the doctor will probably prescribe an NSAID. If swelling is not a problem, he or she may give you acetaminophen.

To avoid drug interactions, overdose, or side effects, make sure that you check with your doctor before taking any over-the-counter medications. (See Chapter 7 for more information on medicines.)

Exercise

If you're in pain, you'll probably want to *stop* moving, and it's certainly advisable for you to rest your joints when you're feeling achy. But too much sitting around can actually be the *worst* thing for you in the long run. Exercise is a great way to "oil and feed" the cartilage. Under-exercised joints don't get the lubricating and nourishing benefits of the in-and-out action of the joint fluid, so cartilage can become thin and dry, losing its resilience and capability to cushion the bones.

You should include three types of exercises in your overall physical fitness program:

- ✔ *Flexibility exercises:* You should do stretching, bending, and twisting exercises every day to increase your range-of-motion and reduce stiffness. Flexibility exercises will help keep your joints loose and flexible.

- ✔ *Strengthening exercises:* Weight lifting or isometric exercises should be done every other day to build your muscles and help keep your joint supporting structures stable. These types of exercises will help increase your muscle strength.

- ✔ *Endurance (aerobic) exercises:* These should be done at least three times a week for at least 20-30 minutes each session to increase overall fitness, strengthen your cardiovascular system, and keep your weight under control. Brisk walking (especially up hills), jogging, cycling, dancing, jumping rope, and so on, will increase your fitness and capacity for exercise.

Before starting a new exercise program, check with your doctor to find out what kinds of exercise and which levels of activity are appropriate for you. Doing the wrong exercises — or doing the right exercises in the wrong way — can cause you further injury. (See Chapter 11 for more information on exercise.)

Joint protection

Learning and applying the techniques of body alignment, proper standing, sitting, walking and running, and correct lifting can go a long way toward sparing your joints from excessive wear-and-tear and protecting them from future injury. You may also find it helpful to wrap affected joints with elastic supports or take a load off with assistive devices, such as canes or crutches, whenever necessary. Other joint-protective techniques include alternating your activities with rest periods, varying your tasks to avoid too much repetitive stress on any one area, and pacing yourself. Don't try to do too much at once. (See Chapter 12 for more information on joint protection.)

Hot and cold packs

Some people prefer heat, others cold, but use whatever works for you. Hot baths, heating pads, electric blankets, and hot tubs can relax painful muscles, while ice packs can numb the affected area. Just make sure you don't use either method for longer than 20 minutes at a time to avoid damaging tissues. (See Chapter 9 for more information on physical therapy for pain relief.)

A good rule to keep in mind is to give your skin time to return to its usual temperature before reapplying hot or cold packs.

Weight control

If you're overweight, your hips, knees, and ankles are probably suffering. Not only are they subjected to a force equal to three times your body weight each time you take a step, they can be pummeled by ten times your body weight if you jog or run! So that extra 10 pounds around your middle may translate to an extra 100 pounds slamming away on certain joints at certain times. And that's only one reason why it's so important to keep your weight at an acceptable level. (See Appendix C for more information on diet and weight control.)

Fifty percent of patients who develop knee osteoarthritis have been overweight for between 3 and 10 years.

Self-help skills

Strategies for pain management, foods and supplements that can help heal, positive thinking, prayer, spirituality, massage, relaxation techniques, and alternative healing methods can add to your arsenal in the fight against pain and disability. Don't ignore their enormous potential to improve the quality of your life. (See Chapters 9, 10, and 14-19 for more information on these topics.)

Surgery

When you have a painful joint that isn't going to get better and the pain is seriously compromising the quality of your life, you may want to consider surgery. These days arthroscopic surgery, cartilage transplants, and joint replacement surgery are routinely performed and can make a huge difference for those who live in pain.(See Chapter 8 for more information on surgery.)

True Patient Story

Mark, a 35-year-old television executive, had been a hotshot college quarterback in his younger days. But after winding up at the bottom of one too many half-ton pileups, his knees were shot.

"I was a sitting duck for those guys," Mark says ruefully. "They just couldn't wait to pounce on me, no matter what the play. After two years of getting hit over and over again, my body just couldn't take it anymore. I was permanently sidelined."

Sidelined from football, perhaps, but not other sports. Over the next several years he took up jogging, karate, fencing, and weight lifting. "I tried to do something every day," Mark said. "But it wasn't just because I wanted to keep in shape. I would literally get itchy if I didn't get a certain amount of exercise on a daily basis." In spite of his efforts, though, he managed to pack an extra 20 pounds onto his once rock-hard body. ("Beer and nachos while watching football," Mark explained, smiling.)

Then one day, right in the middle of a fencing match, his right knee began to hurt. "It was a deep pain, way inside my knee, a pretty intense soreness that lasted through the match and really bugged me," Mark said. Afterward, he iced his knee and the pain went away. But it began to bother him now and again, often during fencing, and also when he was jogging or in the bent-knee stance of karate. When the pain became present more often than not, Mark went to see a sports medicine doctor.

"Sounds to me like osteoarthritis," his doctor said. An X ray confirmed that the cartilage in his knee was "rough" and quite thin. "Arthritis!" Mark exploded. "But that's for old people. I'm only 35!"

Today, two years later, Mark's osteoarthritis is under pretty good control. He rarely has pain, unless he stands in line for long periods of time. And although he has given up certain knee-thrashing sports (such as football, karate, and fencing), he has found that he's still physically able to do just about whatever he wants.

"I chalk my recovery up to two main things," Mark says. "Losing weight and switching activities. Once I dropped that extra 20 pounds I'd been lugging around, my knee pain also dropped about 50 percent. Then I started swimming every day — a real boon to my joints since I could keep them loosened up without the slamming impact of jogging or jumping rope. Yoga has also helped me gain some flexibility while getting rid of some tension. And I've been taking a few supplements that seem to help. All in all, I feel like a brand new guy."

Chapter 3

A War Within: Rheumatoid Arthritis

*R*heumatoid arthritis (RA) is a case of the human body's good intentions gone awry. Your body is equipped with a very effective immune system that fights off bacteria and other foreign bodies. Specialized immune cells attack these invaders, surround them, paralyze them, and destroy them. A strong, intact immune system is absolutely essential to your survival — without it, you would quickly become consumed by infections and disease. But if your immune system should suddenly go haywire and start attacking your body's own tissues, it could become your own worst enemy. Such is the case with rheumatoid arthritis (RA). With RA, the immune system attacks the tissues that cushion and line the joints, eventually causing the entire joint to deteriorate.

This chapter teaches you about the signs and symptoms of RA, the suspected causes, how it's diagnosed and treated, and the difference between rheumatoid arthritis and osteoarthritis.

When the Body Turns on Itself

For reasons that are not completely understood, in rheumatoid arthritis the white blood cells of the immune system attack the joint lining (synovial membrane) as if it were a foreign object. The assaulted membrane becomes inflamed and painful, the entire joint capsule swells, and the synovial cells start to grow and divide in an abnormal way. Almost as if they're launching a counterattack, these abnormal cells invade the surrounding tissue — the bones, cartilage, muscles, and ligaments. The joint space begins to narrow, and the joint's supporting structures become weak. At the same time, the cells that trigger inflammation release enzymes that start eating away at the bone and cartilage, causing joint erosion and scarring. Reeling under this many-sided attack, the joint itself deteriorates, eventually becoming misshapen and misaligned. Pain, loss of movement, and joint destruction are the unhappy results. See Figures 3-1 and 3-2 for comparison.

Rheumatoid arthritis insidiously makes its way through the body and (in more severe cases) can spread to all of the joints, over time. But the joints are not its only targets. RA is a *systemic disease* capable of triggering numerous problems in various parts of the body, not just the joints. It can cause inflammation of the membranes surrounding the eyes, heart, lungs, and other internal organs, generally wreaking havoc.

If the tear and salivary glands partially "dry up," Sjögren's syndrome can develope in assocication with RA. See Chapter 4 for more on this "drying disease."

Some people have RA for just a short time — a few months or a couple of years — and then it disappears forever. Others suffer through painful periods (flares) that come and go, although they can feel quite well in between episodes. Those with severe forms of RA, however, may be in pain a good deal of the time, experience symptoms for many years, and suffer serious joint damage.

Figure 3-1:
In the healthy joint, the synovial membrane is thin and uninflamed; the cartilage is smooth, thick, and even. The joint space is well-defined and the joint capsule assumes a normal shape.

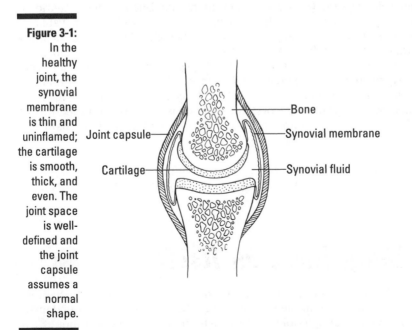

Figure 3-2:
In the joint affected by RA, the synovial membrane is inflamed and swollen, invading both bone and cartilage. The cartilage is thin, the joint space narrowed, and the joint capsule swollen.

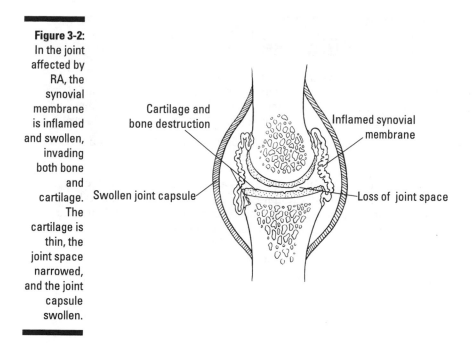

Cartilage and bone destruction

Inflamed synovial membrane

Swollen joint capsule

Loss of joint space

Warning Signs and Symptoms of RA

If you have rheumatoid arthritis, the first thing you may notice is a dull ache, stiffness, and swelling in two matching joints — for example, both elbows, both knees, or both index fingers. The most typical sites for RA are the fingers and wrists, but it can also settle in the hands, elbows, shoulders, neck, hips, knees, ankles, and/or feet. See Figure 3-3.

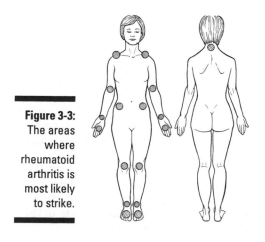

Figure 3-3:
The areas where rheumatoid arthritis is most likely to strike.

Still's disease

Although pain and inflammation are early signs of RA, they're not always the first to herald the arrival of the disease. There's a type of RA, called Still's disease, in which the first indicators are fever, chills, and other general symptoms affecting the entire body, not just the joints. Among children with juvenile rheumatoid arthritis, some 10 percent have Still's disease.

RA typically begins with minor symptoms and slowly makes its presence known. But it can also strike dramatically, causing several joints to become inflamed all at once. Although the symptoms of rheumatoid arthritis vary, most people with RA experience one or more of the following:

- Pain, warmth, redness, swelling, or tightness in a joint
- Joints affected in a symmetrical pattern (for example, both knees, both shoulders, and so on)
- Joint pain or stiffness lasting longer than an hour upon arising or after prolonged inactivity
- Pea-shaped bumps under the skin (called *rheumatoid nodules*), especially on the outside of the elbows, at the base of the scalp, or under the toes
- Evidence of joint erosion on an X ray
- Loss of mobility
- General soreness, aching, stiffness
- A general "sick" feeling (malaise)
- Fatigue and weakness, especially in the early afternoon
- Periodic fever and/or sweats
- Difficulty sleeping
- Anemia
- Blood tests showing the presence of rheumatoid factor (an abnormal substance found in the blood of about 80 percent of RA patients).

As RA progresses, the joints enlarge and can become deformed. They may even freeze in a semi-contracted position, making complete extension impossible. The fingers can start to curl up, pointing away from the thumb, as their tendons slip out of place. If RA should attack the lungs, it can cause *pleurisy* (inflammation of the membranes around the lungs), prompting difficulty in breathing, chest pain, and lung scarring. If it settles in the membrane surrounding the heart (a condition called *pericarditis*), it can cause abnormal heart function. If it affects the blood vessels (*vasculitis*), the blood supply to other parts of the body can be cut off, causing nerve damage and/or tissue death.

Even though rheumatoid arthritis can have some very serious consequences, this disease can be managed. Many people with RA live long, successful lives (See True Patient Story at the end of this chapter.) But remember: Early treatment can make a big difference in RA, so don't wait to see a doctor.

The older you are when rheumatoid arthritis first strikes, the milder your case is likely to be.

What Causes Rheumatoid Arthritis?

The truth is that nobody really knows what causes RA, although it is believed to be linked to a defect in the immune system. Many people with RA have a particular genetic marker — HLA-DR4 — so it's reasonable to suspect that this may be to blame. Yet, not everyone with this gene ends up with RA, and not everyone with RA has this gene. Most likely, genetics *may* play a part in the development of the disease but is not the determining factor. And scientists are certain that more than just one gene is involved: perhaps HLA-DR4 is only one of several genes that can tip the scales in favor of developing RA. Some researchers believe that RA may be triggered by a virus, or perhaps an unrecognized bacteria that "wakes up" a dormant genetic defect and sets it in motion. As of yet, no such infectious agent has been discovered, and RA has not been found to be contagious.

Hormones or hormone deficiencies may also play a part, although it's unclear just what their role may be. Women are more likely then men to develop RA, suggesting a possible link to estrogen. But, at present, there are more questions than answers.

Who Is Most Likely to Get RA?

Rheumatoid arthritis is an equal opportunity disease — just about anybody can get it. Children, the elderly, the middle-aged, and people of almost all racial or ethnic groups can develop RA. Sex is the main determining factor, because the disease tends to favor women, especially those between the ages of 20 and 50. Women, in fact, are two to three times more likely to get RA than men, although scientists have yet to determine why.

Diagnosing Rheumatoid Arthritis

Unfortunately, there isn't any one test that can tell your doctor that you definitely have RA. Instead, he or she will gather information from many sources, looking for a pattern. Diagnosis is based on the information gleaned from a patient's medical history, the physical examination, laboratory tests, X rays, a fluid sample taken from affected joints, and if rheumatoid nodules are present, a biopsy.

Medical history and physical exam

During your initial examination, your doctor will ask about the onset of your symptoms, whether you are experiencing any morning stiffness, the kind and amount of pain you feel, the presence of swelling, whether or not joints are affected on both sides of your body, and so on. The goal in taking the medical history is to see if your symptoms fit the general pattern of RA or suggest another disease instead. He or she will also check for tenderness, range of motion, and the presence of rheumatoid nodules.

Tests

There are three tests typically used to help diagnose rheumatoid arthritis, all of which are done by taking a sample of your blood and sending it to the laboratory for examination. They are the following:

- **Rheumatoid factor (RF) test:** to check for the presence of a particular antibody that appears in the blood of the majority of people who have RA.

- **Erythrocyte sedimentation rate (ESR):** to check for the presence of inflammation in the body.

- **Red blood cell count (RBC):** to check for anemia, a common symptom associated with systemic types of arthritis.

(See Chapter 6 for a complete description of these tests.) In addition to the preceding, your doctor may also perform the following tests:

- **Joint fluid sample:** The doctor may insert a needle into your affected joint(s) to remove some fluid, which will be examined under a microscope for evidence of infection and inflammation.

- **Joint X ray:** An X ray of your joints may be taken to detect early bone and cartilage loss or to serve as a baseline for future X rays.

- **Biopsy of rheumatoid nodules:** If you have rheumatoid nodules, the doctor may want to excise a piece of tissue from one of them and examine it under a microscope to confirm the diagnosis. Here's how it's done: After carefully cleansing the skin and injecting a local anesthetic, the doctor makes a tiny cut near the nodule. If the nodule is easily accessible, the doctor may decide to reach in with a scalpel and shave off a piece of tissue. Or, he or she may push a thin, hollow needle into the nodule and using suction, pull out a sample.

Treating Rheumatoid Arthritis

Although RA is often a chronic disease, most people who have it respond well to treatment and lead active, productive lives. A few years back, a victim of RA could look forward to a dreary life spent bedridden or in a wheelchair. But today, that's rarely the case: Only about one in ten patients progresses to the point of disability. In a full 70 percent of the cases, symptoms are relieved or controlled by treatment for long periods of time. And one out of ten people completely recovers from RA, usually within the first year, never to be bothered by it again.

Treatment usually begins with the least aggressive, most conservative measure, rest, and gradually gives way to more aggressive methods — medication and surgery — if necessary.

Rest

Resting the affected joints during a flare is a must because using them tends to increase inflammation. Regular rest periods should be worked into the daily schedule, and at times, total bed rest may be necessary. Immobilizing a severely affected joint with a splint may help, but the joint should be moved from time to time to keep it from locking up. (See Chapter 9.)

RA appears to be affected by your mental outlook. Stress tends to make flares worse, while a positive outlook can help keep complications at bay.

Diet

You should follow a healthful, nutritious diet, including plenty of fish and plant oils to help reduce inflammation, while avoiding processed meat. (See Chapter 10.)

Physical therapy and exercise

A good overall exercise program will help strengthen joint supporting structures, increase endurance, and maintain or improve flexibility. Even inflamed joints should be exercised a little to prevent them from freezing up. A physical therapist can provide exercises that gently take the joints through their full range of movement. Exercising in water, especially during flares, may be easier than exercising on land, because it's low impact and the cool water may help ease inflammation. (See Chapter 11.)

Joint protection

You should employ techniques for minimizing joint stress through proper body alignment. Maintaining proper posture while walking, standing, and sitting can go a long way toward easing joint stress. And learning how to lift or move heavy objects correctly is also a must. (See Chapter 12.)

Applying hot or cold compresses

If you apply hot or cold packs to inflamed joints, it may ease the pain and help reduce inflammation. Heat is typically used to ease sore muscles and increase circulation, while cold is used to dull the pain and reduce inflammation. (See Chapter 9.)

Medication

Many drugs can be used to combat RA symptoms. The four main types commonly prescribed are in the following sections.

Non-steroidal anti-inflammatory drugs (NSAIDs)

NSAIDs (pronounced n-sayds) reduce swelling, relieve pain, and are the most commonly prescribed drugs for RA. Aspirin and ibuprofen are two well-known NSAIDs, but these drugs are typically prescribed in much larger doses than the over-the-counter brands you can buy at the supermarket. A dose of 325 mg of aspirin taken four times a day is the standard treatment for pain in most newly diagnosed RA patients. (Naturally, you should not take this dosage of aspirin or any other medication unless it is prescribed by your doctor.)

As with all drugs, certain side effects can occur when taking NSAIDs, including upset stomach, nausea, diarrhea, and stomach bleeding. Taking this type of medication with food can help prevent these.

Slow-acting drugs

If NSAIDs aren't effective, or if your disease seems to be progressing quickly, your doctor may want to switch to slow-acting drugs such as gold compounds, penicillamine, or anti-malarial drugs.

Slow-acting drugs are also known as *remittive drugs* and *DMARDs,* which stands for disease-modifying anti-rheumatic drugs. These drugs are called "slow-acting" because it may be weeks or months before results are seen.

These drugs may influence the immune system — whose errant behavior can lead to RA — to slow the formation of bone deformities, affect cell growth, or otherwise slow the progress of RA. They can even send the disease into remission, at least temporarily. Depending upon which drug is being used, it may be given until symptoms improve, until unacceptable side effects appear, or until it's clear that the medicine is not helping.

Potential side effects of DMARDs include gastrointestinal distress (diarrhea, loss of appetite, vomiting, and so on), liver problems, rashes, and blood cell disorders.

Corticosteroids

Corticosteroids, such as prednisone, are powerful weapons against inflammation. They work by suppressing the immune system, which is the trigger of the errant inflammation seen in RA.

These drugs work well because they're "souped up" versions of cortisone, the body's natural immune suppressor. Unfortunately, their effects diminish with time as the body adjusts to them, and they don't to anything to fight the disease itself.

These strong drugs can also trigger severe side effects, including high blood pressure, osteoporosis, an increase in blood glucose, cataracts, as well as bruising and thinning of the skin. When used for a month or longer, they may cause fluid retention in the face ("moon face"), the belly, the legs, and so on. Because of this, corticosteroids are normally prescribed only when severe flares occur or when all other treatments have failed.

If you suddenly stop taking corticosteroids, you may suffer from pain, swelling, and other effects. That's why you should always taper off your use of these drugs.

Immunosuppressive drugs

Used to suppress inflammation and inhibit cell growth, this class of drugs works faster than the slow-acting drugs, and can replace or reduce the use of corticosteroids. Because of their growth-limiting action, certain immunosuppressive drugs (for example, methotrexate, Cytoxan, and Imuran) are also used to treat cancer.

Immunosuppressive drugs can have serious side effects, including liver disease, increased infections, decreased production of blood cells, and lung inflammation. Because of this, their use must be closely monitored by a physician.

Surgery

When all else fails and RA becomes severe or disabling, surgery may be an option. Surgeons have different approaches to relieving the symptoms. Some of the approaches are in the following list:

✔ Diseased joint linings can be surgically removed.

✔ Joint replacement can correct deformities and ease pain.

✔ Fusing or removing joints in the foot may relieve the pain experienced when walking.

✔ Fusing vertebrae in the neck may prevent spinal cord compression.

✔ Fusing of the thumb joint can aid in grasping.

Other sophisticated surgical techniques are on the horizon, assuring people a healthier and more pain-free future.

What's the Difference between Osteoarthritis and Rheumatoid Arthritis?

It would be simpler to explain what these two diseases *do* have in common, namely joint pain and damage to certain joint structures, such as the cartilage and the bone. Other than that, they're about as different as night and day. Table 3-1 outlines the differences between RA and osteoarthritis.

Table 3-1: Rheumatoid Arthritis Compared to Osteoarthritis	
Rheumatoid Arthritis	*Osteoarthritis*
Joint inflammation and swelling are prominent symptoms.	Joint inflammation and swelling are less common.
Usually begins between the ages of 25-50, but can also strike children.	Usually begins after the age of 40. Rarely strikes children.
Settles in a majority of joints, especially fingers, wrists, shoulders, knees, and elbows.	Affects the weight-bearing joints primarily (for example, knees, hips, ankles, and spine).

Rheumatoid Arthritis	Osteoarthritis
Affects joints symmetrically (for example, both wrists).	Affects isolated joints or one joint at a time.
Morning stiffness lasts more than one hour.	Brief periods of morning stiffness.
Often causes the systemic symptoms fatigue, fever, weight loss, and general malaise.	Does not cause systemic symptoms.

Prognosis

It's difficult to predict how a person with RA will fare, because everyone is different. But certain factors can suggest that the course of the disease might be easier or more difficult. For example, RA *may* be less severe if

- ✔ **You are female:** Women are more likely to get RA, but the disease often takes a greater toll on men.
- ✔ **You have a college degree or better:** Educated people tend to seek help earlier, are more likely to follow doctor's orders, have less physically strenuous jobs, and have access to better care.
- ✔ **You are middle-aged or older when stricken.**
- ✔ **Your cartilage and bone ends have not been worn away, and you do not yet have joint deformities.**
- ✔ **You don't have rheumatoid nodules.**
- ✔ **Your level of rheumatoid factor is low.** Remember, however, that some people who have little or no rheumatoid factor suffer severely.
- ✔ **You're pregnant.** Some women enjoy a nine-month period of time with fewer symptoms.

 Perhaps as many as 10 percent of RA patients enjoy what doctors call *spontaneous remission,* or the disappearance of the disease for no apparent reason.

A look at the future

Today, rheumatoid arthritis rarely manifests as the crippling, deforming disease of just a few years ago. Researchers in genetics and immunology are constantly uncovering new and fascinating parts of this puzzle, and some fifteen new drugs have recently been discovered to treat RA. Great strides have also been made in surgical techniques, enabling surgeons to offer hope to those with deformed, painful joints. Through our rapidly expanding arsenal of knowledge, our medications, certain lifestyle changes, and new surgical techniques, we should soon be able to tame, if not conquer, the beast known as rheumatoid arthritis.

True Patient Story

Lucille Ball, the famous comedienne and zany star of the "I Love Lucy" television series, was just 17 years old and working as a model in Hattie Carnegie's internationaly renowned dress shop when she suddenly developed a fiery pain in both her legs. "It was so bad, I had to sit down," she wrote in her autobiography, *Love, Lucy.* She had recently recovered from a bout with pneumonia and a high fever; now this!

Hurrying to her doctor, she received the terrifying news: She had rheumatoid arthritis, a crippling disease that becomes progressively worse over time. In fact, it was conceivable that she would spend her life in a wheelchair. Lucy's doctor sent her to an orthopedic clinic where she waited for three hours, nearly fainting from the pain, before the doctor informed her that there was no cure. He did ask if she would like to try an experimental treatment, though — injections of a kind of "horse serum." Lucy agreed and received these shots over the next several weeks until she finally ran out of money. Unfortunately, the pain continued.

Discouraged but not about to give up, Lucy went back home to her parents, who massaged her legs, gave her money to continue the horse serum injections, and encouraged her to take better care of her health. Finally, months later, the pain began to ease and Lucy was able to stand up on weak and shaky legs. Her left leg had shortened a bit during the course of the disease, so she added a 20-pound weight to her corrective shoe to stretch the leg out.

Lucy's hard work and perseverance paid off. She was able to return to New York; she made several movies and eventually starred in her own television series, one that required vigourus physical comedy, stamina, and energy. She also starred in Broadway plays, performing eight shows a week while managing to sail through energetic song and dance numbers with a seemingly effortless grace and ease. Lucy remained active and healthy until her death in 1989, and in spite of her doctor's ominous prediction, never spent a single day in a wheelchair.

Chapter 4

Other Forms of Arthritis

• •

In This Chapter

▶ Learning about the different forms of arthritis

▶ Understanding various disease processes

▶ Recognizing symptoms

▶ Finding out what doctors can do

▶ Learning what you can do to help yourself

• •

The various forms of arthritis and arthritis-related conditions all have one thing in common: They produce pain, swelling, and/or other problems in or near one or more joints. The symptoms may appear suddenly and obviously, or they might sneak up so gradually that you can't remember when they began. They may strike with the force of a jackhammer or feel more like a chilly breeze. Sometimes the diagnosis is obvious; other times it may elude doctors for a year or longer. The varied treatments can be quick and effective, produce delayed reactions or in some cases, not work at all.

Osteoarthritis and rheumatoid arthritis, the subjects of Chapters 2 and 3, are well-known forms of arthritis. This chapter examines some of the lesser-known and less prevalent, but still troublesome, forms of the disease.

True Arthritis

True arthritis isn't a medical term; it's just a convenient way of referring to the group of ailments in which arthritis is the primary disease process and is a major part of the syndrome. Osteoarthritis and rheumatoid arthritis are the best-known members of this group, which can cause problems ranging from mild joint pain to a bowed permanently spine.

Gout: It's not just for royalty

Many people think that gout is a disease reserved for corpulent kings and beefy barons, but any one of us can be stricken, even if we're slim and never drink alcohol.

Some two million Americans, mostly male, suffer from gout. Officially known as *acute gouty arthritis,* the problem usually begins with a sudden, over-whelming "assault" on a joint. You may go to bed feeling fine, with no inkling of trouble ahead, only to wake up in the middle of the night with excruciating pain in the bunion joint of your big toe. The joint is stiff and warm to the touch; swelling lends a shiny, tight, reddish or purplish look to the skin, which is severely stretched over the area. Sometimes the joint is so inflamed and painful that even the touch of a bed sheet causes agonizing pain. You may also have a fever, chills, a rapid heart rate, and a general "blah" feeling.

The big toe is quite often the first site that gout strikes. The elbows, wrists, fingers, knees, ankles, heels, and instep may also be attacked during the first or subsequent bouts, while the shoulders, spine, and hips are rarely touched.

No matter where gout strikes first, the odds are 3 out of 4 that it will get to the big toe at some point.

Your first attack of gout may also be your last, for gout often disappears in several days without treatment and without lingering after effects. Or, it may herald the beginning of a series of attacks on that joint and/or others, leading to progressive and irreversible joint injury. Fortunately, medical treatment can help ward off recurring attacks while preventing or minimizing perma-nent joint damage.

What causes gout?

Gout is linked to excess uric acid in the blood. (Doctors call this *hyper-uricemia.*) When the blood has more uric acid than it can handle, the body may convert the excess into sharp, pointed crystals and store them in one or more joints. See Figure 4-1 for an example of what the crystal deposits look like in a joint.

If you want to guard against gout, the best strategy is probably to be born female. Women's uric acid levels are lower than men's up until menopause. After menopause, women's uric acid levels start to rise, but up to twenty years may pass before they are equal to male levels.

Several situations can lead to an excessive amount of uric acid, including the following:

✔ Genetics (6-18 percent of those with gout have the disease in the family).

✔ Eating lots of organ meat and/or other meats, gravies, peas, anchovies, dried peas and beans. These foods contain large amounts of purines that can stimulate the body's production of uric acid.

✔ Blood cancer or other diseases that cause the rapid multiplication and destruction of body cells, leading to higher levels of purines and uric acid.

✔ Certain diseases that hamper the kidneys' capability to filter out uric acid.

✔ Drinking too much alcohol (which can upset kidney function).

✔ Taking drugs that can lead to increased uric acid.

Gout comes about when excess uric acid in the blood is converted into crystalline form and deposited in the joints. But elevated uric acid by itself does not cause gout — many people with excess uric acid suffer nary a twinge, while others, with terrible pain, have fairly standard amounts of uric acid. You can also have fully formed uric acid crystals in a joint or two, yet feel no pain.

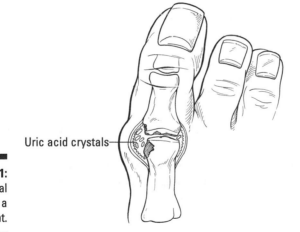

Uric acid crystals

Figure 4-1:
Crystal
deposits in a
gouty joint.

Diagnosing and treating gout

Sometimes the symptoms of gout "speak" loudly, making the diagnosis fairly easy. Other times, the symptoms can be vague, making the diagnosis difficult.

Microscopic examination of fluid taken from the stricken joint is an important diagnostic step. If needle-like uric acid crystals are visible, it's most likely gout. White blood cells may also be present, sent to the joint as part of the inflammation process. The doctor will order a blood test to check uric acid levels, x-ray the afflicted joint and look for *tophi* (lumps of uric acid crystals stored under the skin).

There is no absolute cure for gout, although there are helpful medications and lifestyle changes. Treatment often begins with high doses of non-steroidal anti-inflammatory drugs (NSAIDs) for pain and inflammation, and costicosteroids may be injected into the afflicted joint. A drug called colchicine is helpful, although you must start using it soon after gout strikes for it to be effective. NSAIDs and colchicines may be given to prevent further attacks. If that doesn't work, you may be given drugs such as allupurinol and probenecid to keep your uric acid levels under control.

In addition to offering medicines, your doctor can "tap" your joint by inserting a needle and drawing out the excess fluid. This often helps relieve the pain and pressure, and sometimes it's all that's needed.

What you can do

You can help heal gout and prevent its recurrence by doing the following:

- ✔ Losing weight if you are overweight
- ✔ Eliminating alcohol intake
- ✔ Eliminating foods containing purines (for example, organ meats, fatty meats, meat gravies, wild game, sardines, anchovies, herring, mackerel, and scallops) and limiting meat, fish, poultry, dried peas, and beans to one serving per day
- ✔ Working with your doctor to keep your blood pressure under control, if it's a problem
- ✔ Consulting with your doctor to make sure you're not taking any medicines or supplements that encourage gout or interfere with your treatment
- ✔ Exercising regularly

Pseudogout — the royal pretender

Where gout is an ancient disease that ruined many a medieval VIP's days, pseudogout is a "new" affliction. Although it's probably been around as long as "regular" gout, doctors didn't realize it was a separate problem until about

40 years ago. The symptoms of pseudogout are similar to those of gout, but there are no needle-like uric acid crystals in the joint. Instead, there are rhomboid-shaped crystals made up of calcium pyrophosphate dihydrate.

Causes of pseudogout

The causes of pseudogout are unknown. It may be touched off by surgery, a hormonal imbalance, or a metabolic upset. Sometimes it strikes in conjunction with other diseases or states, such as low blood magnesium or too much iron in body tissues. Pseudogout strikes men and women at about the same rate and prefers older folk, especially those over the age of 60.

Symptoms are similar to those seen with gout, but are not consistent from patient to patient. The disease may be acute or chronic. The acute attacks are likely to strike suddenly, settle in the knee, and last for several days. (Fortunately, they are not as painful as acute attacks of "true" gout.) The chronic attacks typically target more than one joint at once. Over time, chronic pseudogout can severely damage joints.

Diagnosing and treating pseudogout

Because pseudogout can masquerade as gout, rheumatoid arthritis, or other ailments, diagnosis is usually made by inspecting fluid taken from the affected joint. If you have pseudogout, your fluid will contain calcium pyrophosphate dihydrate crystals. (These crystals can also be picked up on X rays.)

Unfortunately, there's no way to cure the disease completely and no method for removing the offending crystals from the joints. Instead, doctors try to relieve the symptoms, typically prescribing NSAIDs to reduce the pain and inflammation. Other drugs may be used if necessary. Sometimes, simply "tapping" the joint and drawing out the excess fluid is enough. Treatment can bring relief during attacks but cannot prevent joint damage. Still, most sufferers do well if their pain and inflammation is kept under control by medication.

Juvenile rheumatoid arthritis

Arthritis is bad for everyone, but somehow it seems worse when it strikes children. Youngsters can develop most of the forms that strike adults, and some 280,000 have done so. Many of them suffer from juvenile rheumatoid arthritis (JRA).

To be considered JRA, the disease must produce joint inflammation and stiffness for at least six weeks in someone under the age of 17. JRA is similar to "adult" rheumatoid arthritis, but there are a few key differences:

✔ Many children with JRA outgrow the problem, while most adults with RA do not.

✔ JRA may affect bone development and growth in children, causing slow, rapid, or uneven growth in the afflicted joints.

✔ Less than 50 percent of those with JRA are positive for rheumatoid arthritis factor, compared to 70 or 80 percent of adults.

There are three kinds of juvenile rheumatoid arthritis, differentiated by their symptoms:

✔ **Pauciarticular JRA:** The most common form of JRA, pauciarticular JRA, involves no more than four joints. About 50 percent of children with JRA have pauciarticular JRA, which usually strikes in the knees and other large joints, attacks girls age 8 and younger, and may only strike one of a pair of joints (one knee rather than both, one elbow instead of both, and so on). In 20-30 percent of cases, pauciarticular JRA can trigger eye inflammation that if untreated, can become serious. Fortunately, many children outgrow this disease (although the eye problems can continue into adulthood).

✔ **Polyarticular JRA:** Polyarticular JRA attacks five or more joints. Striking some 30 percent of children with JRA, the polyarticular form usually settles in the fingers and other small joints, although large joints are not immune. The disease is typically symmetrical, which means it attacks the fingers on both hands, and so on. There may also be a fever and rheumatoid nodules. Girls are more likely than boys to develop polyarticular JRA.

✔ **Systemic JRA:** The systemic form of JRA "travels" throughout bodily systems, causing trouble wherever it settles. The least common form of juvenile rheumatoid arthritis, systemic JRA may produce fever, pale red spots on various parts of the body, anemia, swollen lymph nodes, inflammation of the linings of the lungs and heart, and other problems.

Regardless of the form JRA takes, it causes joint stiffness, pain, and swelling that is usually worse upon awakening from a nap or full night's sleep. Symptoms usually come and go. Sometimes a child is lucky: The symptoms arise just a few times, then disappear forever.

Doctors diagnose and treat JRA in much the same way they do the adult version. In addition to the strict medical treatment, children with JRA need special emotional and social support.

Infectious arthritis: When "regular" viruses, bacteria, and fungi invade the joints

Infectious arthritis is caused by viruses, bacteria, or fungi that enter the body and settle into one or more joints. Depending upon which germs have invaded, which joint(s) they inhabit, the strength of your immune system, and the speed and accuracy of the treatment, a bout with infectious arthritis can be brief and relatively painless or serious and painful.

Technically speaking, infectious arthritis is an infection of the joint tissues and/or fluid. Several different germs, ranging from staphylococci to HIV to tuberculosis can infect a joint. But remember, these are not specifically "arthritis germs," they are " regular germs" that cause staph infections, mumps, hepatitis B, and other diseases. It's only when they settle in the joints that infectious arthritis can occur.

The nature and extent of the symptoms depend on which germ has taken up residence in the joint(s). In the joint itself, there may be pain to the touch or with movement, as well as swelling and stiffness. The skin around the joint may be red and puffy. If the infection spreads beyond the joint, there may also be fever and other symptoms. Some forms of infectious arthritis can hit strong and fast, so it's important that you see your doctor immediately if you have any symptoms. If left untreated, they may seriously damage joints within just a few days or weeks.

If your doctor suspects infectious arthritis, he or she will quickly call for various tests to firm up the diagnosis. Blood, urine, and joint fluid samples will be analyzed for infectious organisms. But even before the lab results come back, your doctor may begin giving you antibiotics, starting with those that kill the "usual suspects." Other medicines may follow after the doctor is sure what's ailing you.

Antibiotics are effective against bacterial infections, and antifungal medicines fight fungus infections, but viruses are another story. There are, unfortunately, no effective antiviral medications. But don't despair if you have a virus; many viruses clear up on their own.

In addition to the medicines, your doctor may drain pus from your joint, splint the joint, if necessary, and arrange for physical therapy.

Gonococcal arthritis — an unpleasant side effect

Caused by the *gonococci* bacterium — the same culprit responsible for gonorrhea — gonococcal arthritis is the most widespread of the infectious forms of arthritis. Gonococcal arthritis typically strikes hard and fast, and pain seems to move from one joint to another. Small blisters can appear on the skin over some or many parts of the body, and the tendons may swell and ache.

Both men and women can develop gonococcal arthritis. Men are much more likely to know that something is wrong because of penile discharge and painful urination. Thus, they are more likely to receive treatment for gonorrhea before it progresses to gonococcal arthritis. Women, who don't have such obvious symptoms, are less likely to receive early treatment for gonorrhea and more likely to develop the arthritis. Women may also find themselves suffering from pain in the abdomen and fever.

The typical patient with this disease is a young, sexually active person with signs and symptoms of venereal disease, so the doctor can often home in on the diagnosis of gonococcal arthritis during the history and physical examination. He checks for skin blisters and sends samples of various body fluids to the laboratory before making a definitive diagnosis.

Treatment with antibiotics is usually successful and in most cases, the disease vanishes without permanently damaging the joints.

Psoriatic arthritis — from psoriasis to arthritis

Psoriatic arthritis is an "insult added to the injury" of psoriasis, because it strikes those who are already suffering from this scaly skin condition. Fortunately, only about five percent of psoriasis sufferers develop the arthritis, in which the joints of the fingers and toes become inflamed, swollen, and, in more severe cases, deformed. The spine, hips, and other joints may suffer as well.

There is no specific test for psoriatic arthritis, so your doctor will base the diagnosis on your symptoms, and to some extent, your family medical history. (If you have psoriasis in your family, you're more likely to develop psoriatic arthritis.)

Treatment is important, because psoriatic arthritis can cause severe damage to your joints. Unfortunately, there is no cure. Your doctor will try to reduce your joint inflammation and keep your psoriasis under control. He may pre-scribe methotrexate, fulfasalazine, etretinate, gold compounds, and other drugs to help.

Ankylosing spondylitis — when the spine stiffens

Have you ever seen someone walking bent forward at the waist, back straight, and practically parallel to the ground like Groucho Marx? More likely than not, that person had ankylosing spondylitis (AS).

AS attacks the cartilage, ligaments, and tendons of the spine, which become inflamed. The back becomes stiff, inflamed, and sore. As the disease pro-gresses, the ligaments and tendons may become more like bone tissue, forming bony bridges between the vertebrae and locking them into place. In more severe cases, AS can turn the spine into an unbending rod, but fortu-nately the disease usually doesn't advance that far. Figure 4-2 shows the difference between a normal spine and one with AS.

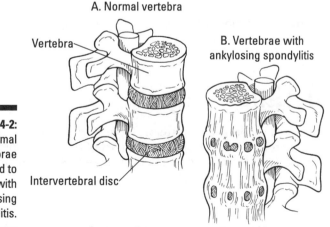

A. Normal vertebra

Vertebra

B. Vertebrae with ankylosing spondylitis

Figure 4-2: Normal vertebrae compared to those with ankylosing spondylitis.

Intervertebral disc

AS has attacked some 300,000 Americans, with men between the ages of 20 and 40 being the favorite targets. The disease has been linked to a certain gene and often runs in families. But having the gene does not guarantee that you will get AS. It increases your susceptibility, but something else, perhaps an infection, must trigger the disease.

AS generally comes on gradually. Pain or stiffness settles in the lower back or other joints. It may be worse at night or upon arising, then get better as the person begins to move around. It can be fairly constant or come and go. Problems may also develop with the shoulders, hips, knees, and other joints.

A systemic disease, AS can cause skin and eye problems, loss of appetite, fatigue, and fever. There may also be difficulty in taking a deep breath, damage to the heart valves, and problems caused by pressure on the nerves.

There isn't any one test that can detect ankylosing spondylitis, so doctors usually make the diagnosis on the basis of the patient's symptoms and family history, plus the physical examination. Your doctor will have you perform various bending exercises to test joint flexibility and will take an X ray to look for characteristic bone damage. He or she will order certain laboratory tests to rule out rheumatoid arthritis or other diseases.

Treatment is aimed at relieving pain and inflammation and preventing or corzrecting deformities of the spine and other problems. Your doctor will typically prescribe NSAIDs and muscle relaxants. Although there's no way to undo the damage that caused the spinal deformities, exercises can help you remain as strong and flexible as possible. Physical therapy can be helpful as you learn to cope with any deformities that arise. More extreme cases may require surgical replacement of a joint.

There is no cure for AS, but most with the disease have only modest to middling symptoms and do fairly well.

Arthritis as a Major Player

In ailments such as scleroderma and systemic lupus erythematosus, the joint problems that characterize arthritis are a major part of the syndrome. But even though arthritis is present — often in a big way — it is not the primary disease process.

Systemic lupus erythematosus — the wolf disease

Systemic lupus erythematosus (commonly known as *lupus* or *SLE*) is a body-wide disease that often marks its victims with a red, wolf-like facial rash.

Lupus can attack the joints, heart, nervous and vascular systems, skin, lungs, and other parts of the body. The symptoms strike because the body produces large numbers of antibodies — called *autoantibodies* — that attack bodily tissue. No one knows exactly why this occurs.

Ninety percent of lupus patients are women, and most of them are in their childbearing years. Perhaps as many as two million Americans suffer from the disease, which tends to favor African-Americans and Hispanics over Caucasians.

Symptoms

Symptoms can range from mild to deadly, with problems appearing in the joints, skin, organs, and/or elsewhere. Typical symptoms include fever, the "blahs," joint pain and inflammation — in other words, arthritis — rash, hair loss, excessive sensitivity to sunlight, anemia, immune system weakness, problems with the kidneys and other organs, nervous system disorders, and depression.

Lupus settles in for the long haul but tends to hit and run, causing symptoms to flare up, then retreat. For many people, the "good" periods can last for weeks, months, or even years.

Diagnosing and treating lupus

Lupus can cause a bewildering variety of symptoms that may mirror those of other diseases, making the diagnosis difficult. Doctors sometimes follow a hunch, tying the fact that the patient is a young woman to one or more of her symptoms, then ordering tests to confirm or rule out the diagnosis. Blood tests are used to look for antibody abnormalities, abnormal blood chemistries, problems with the immune system, kidney damage, and so on. Biopsies of the kidneys, lungs, and other tissues may be required, as well as X rays, CAT scans, MRIs, electrocardiograms, and more.

Treatment is as varied as the disease. In mild cases, the main thrust may center on relieving symptoms: NSAIDs for arthritis symptoms and fever, aspirin to prevent unnecessary blood clots, other drugs for skin problems, and so on. More severe cases may require prednisone or other corticosteroids to bring down inflammation, immunosuppressives to keep the haywire immune system in check, and antimalarial medications for both skin and joint problems.

What you can do

The good news is that there are several things you can do to cope with lupus. You can't make the symptoms disappear, but you can certainly improve the quality of your life by doing the following:

✔ If you tire easily, cut back on your work or home duties.

✔ Look for ways to reduce stress. (See Chapter 15 for tips on coping with stress.)

✔ Protect yourself from the sun.

✔ Follow your doctor's dietary instructions carefully.

Discoid lupus erythematosus: A less dangerous form

A limited form of the disease, discoid lupus generally confines itself to the skin and usually does not venture into the body to attack the organs.

Like systemic lupus, it tends to attack women and produces a characteristic skin rash. The rash begins with little, reddish, disc-like patches, about as big around as the circumference of a drinking straw. Typically appearing on the face, scalp, and ears, they may also appear on the upper chest and back, the backs of the arms, and even the shins. Untreated, the rashes may begin to grow outward and a scar may develop in the central area of each rash. Over time, there can be severe scarring and pitting of the skin, as well as hair loss.

The rash can come and go, or remain in place, and it may be accompanied by joint aches. A drop in the white blood cell count, indicating immune system depression, is also common.

Discoid lupus is difficult to diagnosis because the primary symptom — the rash — can lead doctors to suspect SLE, seborrheic dermatitis, and other diseases. Because there is no single, conclusive test for discoid lupus, much of the diagnostic workup is aimed at eliminating other diseases, then diagnosing discoid lupus by default.

Treatment usually consists of administering corticosteroids, either tablets or cream, which are applied directly to the rash. More serious cases may also require drugs to suppress the errant immune system. If the disease is detected and treated early, scarring can be kept to a minimum.

From wolves to butterflies

Today we think the characteristic SLE rash looks more like a butterfly with its wings spread, but the French doctor who gave the disease its name back in the 1800s thought of a wolf when he saw the rash. The name *lupus,* which means wolf in Classical Latin, has endured.

Scleroderma — when the skin hardens

Although it attacks various parts of the body, scleroderma is best known for its effects on the skin. In fact, the disease's name comes from the Greek words for *hard* and *skin*.

Technically speaking, scleroderma is a collagen vascular disease: *collagen* because an excessive deposition of collagen damages body tissue, and *vascular* because the blood vessels suffer.

No one knows why, but in the 50,000 to 100,000 Americans who have scleroderma, the body produces too much collagen. A fibrous material found in cartilage, skin, and bones, *collagen* is a structural material.

Unable to dispose of the excess collegen properly, the body starts storing it in body tissues in harmful ways. Too much collagen in the skin, for example, makes the skin tight and hard; too much in the organs makes it difficult — if not impossible — for them to work. To make matters worse, the cells in the lining of the blood vessels begin to grow abnormally. With these vital delivery and waste roads hampered, the body has even more difficulty operating effectively.

We don't know exactly why scleroderma develops. Immune system errors are a likely candidate. Hormonal upsets are also possible culprits, and this would explain why women are much more likely to get the disease than men.

Symptoms and progression

The symptoms of scleroderma vary from person to person. It often begins with joint pain, but sometimes the first symptom is difficulty swallowing. It may progress rapidly and fatally, or it may confine itself to the skin for years or decades before moving on to attack other parts of the body. Symptoms of scleroderma include:

- **Skin problems:** Thickening, hardening, roughness, and/or dryness of the skin on the fingers, arms, face, and elsewhere. There may also be "spider veins" on the face, tongue, chest, and fingers, as well as lumpy calcium deposits under the skin.

- **Joint pain, swelling, and "locking":** Pain in the joints can make scleroderma appear to be rheumatoid arthritis. As the disease advances, the elbows, wrists, and fingers may become locked in a closed position.

- **Difficulty swallowing:** If collagen is deposited in the esophagus there may be trouble swallowing.

> ✔ **Digestive difficulties:** If the intestines are strewn with collagen, there may be trouble digesting food and absorbing nutrients.
>
> ✔ **Raynaud's phenomenon:** Many scleroderma patients develop this extreme sensitivity to cold in the fingers and/or toes.

Scleroderma patients can also suffer from a host of other problems, depending upon which organs are overrun with collagen. If the heart is involved, for example, symptoms can range from irregular heartbeat to heart failure.

Diagnosing and treating scleroderma

Diagnosing scleroderma can be difficult in the early stages, especially if joint pain and tenderness are the only symptoms. Once skin changes or difficulty swallowing become apparent, the identification process is much easier.

After a history and physical examination, the doctor will call for special X rays to check the esophagus and gastrointestinal system, blood tests to assess lung function, a skin biopsy to search for excess collagen, and other tests to measure the extent of the problem.

There is no cure for scleroderma, but there are drugs for the various symptoms, including NSAIDs for pain and inflammation, antihypertensives to lower elevated blood pressure, antacids and histamine-blockers for heartburn, and so on. Surgery may be necessary if the disease triggers a severe case of heartburn, while exercise and physical therapy can help strengthen muscles and "oil" the affected joints.

What you can do

Although there are no "home cures" for scleroderma, there are several things you can do to help relieve the problems it produces and improve the quality of your life:

> ✔ Help protect your skin by limiting yourself to short showers or baths, keeping it moist with creams and lotions, and avoiding strong soaps and household chemicals.
>
> ✔ Use a humidifier if indoor heaters are drying out your skin.
>
> ✔ Diligently perform the flexibility and strengthening exercises that your doctor or physical therapist prescribes. The exercises may be difficult to do, but they will help you maintain joint function.
>
> ✔ If swallowing is difficult, chew your food well, avoid foods that are hard to swallow, and drink plenty of liquids with your meals.

> ✔ If nighttime heartburn is a problem, use extra pillows to elevate your head. You can get the same effect by placing blocks under the legs of the bed frame at the head of the bed. Also, try eating dinner earlier than usual or having a light meal so there's less in your stomach at bedtime.

The symptoms of scleroderma are daunting and there is no way to stop the over-active collagen "factories." Still, many people do well for years or even decades, especially if the disease first manifests in the joints and skin rather than in the organs.

Reiter's syndrome: from a stomachache to arthritis

Like gonococcal arthritis, Reiter's syndrome can stem from a venereal infection. But Reiter's is not necessarily the unhappy result of unprotected sex. It can also develop after an intestinal infection — and sometimes seems to strike without an infectious prelude. Reiter's has three classic groups of symptoms: arthritis, conjunctivitis, and urethritis as follows:

> ✔ **Arthritis** takes the form of mild to severe pain and inflammation, often in the feet, ankles, and knees. The wrists, fingers, and other joints may also be struck. The arthritis may vanish or return episodically for years.
>
> ✔ **Conjunctivitis** is an inflammation of the mucous membranes protecting the eyelid and eyeball, causing them to become red and swollen, to burn, itch, and water excessively.
>
> ✔ **Urethritis** is an inflammation of the *urethra*, the "pipe" that conducts urine from the bladder to the outside of the body.

In addition, there may be thick, crusty rashes on the soles of the feet or the palms of the hands, sores in the mouth or vagina and on the tongue or penis, yellowish deposits under the fingernails and toenails, and problems with the heart. Men age 20-50 are the most likely group to be struck.

Young men are more likely to get Reiter's syndrome than any other form of arthritis. Three percent of all men who have a sexually transmitted disease will also be struck by Reiter's.

Chlamydia trachomatis is the bacteria responsible for the largest number of Reiter's cases associated with sexual contact. As for Reiter's linked to gastrointestinal infection, the major culprits are campylobacter, salmonella, shigella, and yersinia.

The diagnosis of Reiter's can be difficult and delayed, for there is no single symptom or definitive test to rely on. The presence of the three classic symptoms is an important clue, but they may not appear at the same time. Doctors generally send samples of a patient's joint fluid plus samples "swabbed" from the urethra to the laboratory for analysis.

Part of the diagnostic workup is designed to rule out other diseases such as lupus and rheumatoid arthritis, while other parts are designed to "rule in" Reiter's. For example, finding the HLA-B27 gene and the presence of an infectious agent such as *Chlamydia* increases the likelihood of Reiter's. X rays showing damage to the cartilage or bone, bony deposits where the bones and tendons meet, soft tissue swelling, and other signs also point to Reiter's syndrome.

Your doctor will prescribe antibiotics to treat the infection and NSAIDs for the arthritis symptoms. He may also prescribe stronger drugs, such as corticosteroids or immunosuppressives. The conjunctivitis is not usually treated directly, although patients may be given eye drops or an ointment for symptomatic relief. Bed rest and exercise are also helpful.

The outlook is generally good for Reiter's patients. Many recover substantially within 5 or 6 months, although mild to moderate arthritis may linger. About a fifth of all patients wind up with chronic, generally mild arthritis, and only a small percentage suffer from severe, on-going symptoms and joint deformity.

Lyme disease — when you're in the bull's-eye

This new version of arthritis popped up during the 1970's in the town of Lyme, Connecticut. Local doctors were puzzled when individuals, groups of friends, and even entire families began developing a disease that looked a lot like arthritis, but didn't fall into any of the known categories.

Fortunately, doctors realized that more people developed the disease during the summer than in any other time of the year, that many patients had developed a large, round "bull's-eye" rash, and that the town of Lyme was surrounded by wooded areas harboring deer and other wild animals. By putting these and other facts together, they discovered that they were looking at a new disease caused by a bacteria called *borrelia burdgorferi,* which was carried by certain ticks who were hitching rides on deer in the nearby woods. When these ticks bit people, the bacteria was passed into their bodies. (And you needn't go into the woods to contract Lyme disease — your dog or cat can bring the offending ticks into your home.)

The first symptom of Lyme disease is likely a large red spot on your rear end, thigh, trunk, or armpit. The rash may have a "blank" spot area in the center, making it look like a bull's-eye. It may itch and be painful or hot.

About half of those with untreated Lyme's disease develop recurrent attacks of arthritis, which manifest as swelling and pain in the knees and other joints, including the shoulders, elbows, wrists, and ankles. These arthritis attacks may last for several months. Unfortunately, up to 20 percent may go on to suffer from chronic arthritis.

Other common symptoms include fever, fatigue, chills, joint pain, muscle aches, headache, and stiff neck. Less common are a sore throat, swollen lymph nodes, nausea, vomiting, backaches, and other problems. These early symptoms may come and go. There may also be nerve disorders, memory deficits and difficult concentrating, heart and liver problems, skin disorders, fatigue, and eye inflammation.

Diagnosing and treating Lyme disease

The diagnosis is made from a combination of the patient's personal history, the physical examination, and results of the laboratory tests. The patient's history is a very important part of the diagnostic procedure. Knowing that the patient went hiking in the woods and that the problems began in the summer, for example, are significant clues.

The key blood test looks for the presence of antibodies to *borrelia burdgorferi*. In patients with nervous system disorders, doctors may perform a spinal tap to look for the antibodies in the spinal fluid. Unfortunately, antibodies don't show up right away, so it may be a while before a definitive diagnosis can be made.

Arresting the spread of Lyme disease is often fairly easy if treatment is started early. Antibiotics, taken orally or given intravenously, can often halt its progress and prevent the appearance of arthritis and other later-stage symptoms. More severe cases can require treatment with IV antibiotics for several weeks. In some people, years may pass before all the symptoms finally vanish.

The doctor may also prescribe NSAIDs for pain and swelling, as well as crutches or other specific treatments or aids, depending on the part of the body affected.

What you can do

The key is to make your body a "tick-free zone." If you go into the woods or other areas where there are deer or other wild animals, you should remember precautions:

✔ Use insect repellent.

✔ Use your clothing as a shield over exposed areas of skin.

✔ Wear light-colored clothes so the dark-colored ticks will stand out if they get on you.

✔ Walk on trails if possible, especially in the center of the trails, giving a wide berth to ticks in the grass and brush.

✔ Admire any animals you come across from a distance.

✔ Afterwards, carefully check yourself and your children for ticks. Pay special attention to the hairy areas of the body.

✔ If you live in a tick-invested area or near the woods, make sure your pets have flea and tick collars.

✔ Watch for the tell-tale bull's-eye spot on your trunk, rear end, or thighs, or in your armpit. If you find one, see your doctor immediately.

Fortunately, the outlook is good for those with Lyme disease, especially if it's caught and treated early.

Arthritis As a Minor Player

Arthritis may appear in bursitis, polymyalgia rheumatica, and the other diseases in this category, but the arthritis is a minor part of the syndrome.

Bursitis: When the sacs become swollen

Bursa are little, fluid-filled sacs strategically placed throughout the body. They're designed to help reduce the friction caused by movement in the joints. Unfortunately, the bursa can become inflamed if injured or overused. This inflammation can also be prompted by infections or certain forms of arthritis, such as gout. When one or more *bursae* becomes inflamed, you have bursitis. The normally flat sacs swell with excess fluid, producing pain and often limiting movement. The shoulders are common targets of bursitis; the elbows, joints of the foot, and other joints can also be struck. See Figure 4-3 for an example of where the bursa are located in the shoulder.

The pain and resulting movement limitation can range from mild to severe. You may have a nagging little pain in one hip or such severe shoulder pain that dressing is difficult.

There are no tests for bursitis. Instead, the doctor must rely on the patient's history and symptoms, as well as a physical examination of the affected areas to make the diagnosis. She or he may also draw some fluid out of the bursa to try to determine the cause of the inflammation.

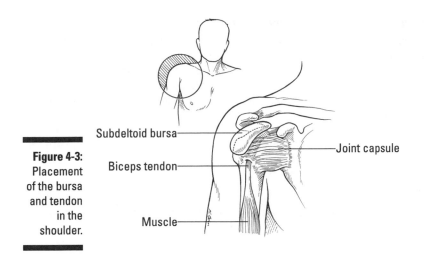

Figure 4-3:
Placement
of the bursa
and tendon
in the
shoulder.

Subdeltoid bursa

Joint capsule

Biceps tendon

Muscle

In many cases, treatment is limited to pain pills, rest, and perhaps joint immo-bilization. If the bursa is infected, the doctor may drain it and give you antibiotics. For chronic and severe bursitis, prednisone or another corticos-teroid may be required. Exercise can help restore the range of motion and rebuild weakened muscles.

Tendonitis/Tenosynovitis: Inflammation of bone and muscle attachments

When certain muscles contract or relax, our bones move accordingly. But the bone-and-muscle, contract-and-relax-system depends on the connecting link: the tendons, which join muscle to bone.

Tendons are the tough, fibrous extensions at the ends of the muscles that attach themselves to the bones. *Tendonitis* occurs when one or more of these tendons become inflamed. Most often associated with repetitive motions, impingements, strenuous activity, and advancing years, this ailment can leave tendons red, raw, and painful to the touch or upon movement.

The sheaths surrounding the tendons may also become inflamed, producing a condition known as *tenosynovitis*. If the sheaths dry out and rub against the tendon, they produce a grating sound or sensation. Various diseases, includ-ing scleroderma, gout, and gonorrhea can cause tenosynovitis.

Diagnosing and treating tendonitis/tenosynovitis

The diagnosis will be based on your symptoms, medical history, and the physical examination. Your doctor may prescribe medications such as NSAIDs to counteract pain and inflammation. Corticosteroids or local anesthetics are sometimes injected right into the sheath surrounding the tendon. Chronic problems may require surgery to remove calcium deposits or release contracted tendons.

The outlook for those with tendonitis/tenosynovitis is good, and the problem often clears up on it own.

What you can do

There are a few easy, inexpensive ways to help alleviate the pain. You may want to try the following:

- Stop the activity that caused the inflammation
- Rest
- Apply hot or cold packs to the area
- Immobilize the involved joints

Raynaud's phenomenon/disease: A chilling problem

The hallmark of Raynaud's is discoloration, tingling, burning, pain and/or numbness in one or more fingers or toes, and less commonly, the nose, lips, or ear lobes. Spasms of the small arteries that supply blood to these areas cause these symptoms by diminishing the blood supply. Brought on by cold temperatures and/or emotional stress, these spasms can last a few minutes or go on for hours. Chronic Raynaud's can lead to skin changes, as well as sores on the ends of the toes and fingers.

Raynaud's comes in two forms:

- **Raynaud's disease:** Also known as Primary Raynaud's, this is the more common form. Typically a milder version of the problem, it acts alone when it attacks.
- **Raynaud's phenomenon:** Also known as Secondary Raynaud's, this is less common. The more serious form of the ailment, it is brought on by another disease or condition such as scleroderma or lupus.

Certain types of work increase a person's vulnerability to Raynaud's. Those who operate vibrating tools, who are exposed to vinyl chloride, and who type, play the piano, or otherwise subject their fingers to repetitive stress are more likely to develop this problem.

Diagnosing and treating Raynaud's

Diagnosing Raynaud's can be easy, but distinguishing one form from the other can be more problematic. Diagnosis and differentiation is made on the basis of the person's symptoms and laboratory tests, such as the antinuclear antibody test and erythrocyte sedimentation rate. Much of the laboratory testing is done to rule out other diseases. One test, the nail fold capillaroscopy, can help separate Raynaud's disease from Raynaud's phenomenon.

Treatment for Raynaud's may be as simple as teaching patients what they can do for themselves and monitoring the situation, or it may include powerful drugs. In very severe cases, nerves to the afflicted areas may be cut to provide temporary relief.

What you can do

Your Raynaud's may be here to stay, but you needn't be a helpless victim. You can fight back in several ways:

- ✔ Stay warm all over. (Dress warmly, layer your clothing, and wear absorbent socks and underwear to draw perspiration away from your skin.)

- ✔ Immerse your fingers and toes in warm water to help keep them warm.

- ✔ If you smoke, stop. (Nicotine constricts blood vessels, a major problem with Raynaud's.)

- ✔ Speak to your doctor about the possibility of switching medicines if you are taking beta-blockers or other drugs that constrict blood vessels.

- ✔ Learn to control your reaction to stress.

- ✔ Exercise regularly.

Sjögren's syndrome: dry mouth, eyes, and maybe more

No one knows what causes this disease, but it's clear that the immune system is involved. The characteristic dryness in the mouth and eyes occurs when those mainstays of the immune system, the white blood cells, invade and damage the salivary and tear glands. The same problem can also cause dryness of the trachea, vagina, the lining of the gastrointestinal tract, and other parts of the body.

About one-third of Sjögren's sufferers develop an arthritis similar to rheumatoid arthritis, but usually less severe.

There's an interesting link between Sjögren's and a cancer called lymphoma: those with this "drying syndrome" are more than 40 times more likely to develop lymphoma than people who do not have Sjögren's.

The combination of dry mouth, dry eyes, and joint distress can make diagnosis a simple matter. Tests can confirm that the level of tears and saliva production is sub par. Further clues can be found in the abnormal blood tests. Antibody abnormalities and possibly anemia, fewer white blood cells, and an elevated erythrocyte sedimentation rate may be found.

Sjögren's syndrome cannot be cured, but many of the symptoms can be alleviated. By chewing gum, sipping fluid, using a mouth rinse and artificial tear drops, you can help keep your eyes and mouth moist. A drug called pilocarpine may be given to increase the production of saliva. Pain and swelling of the salivary glands and joints can be treated with painkillers, but stronger drugs may be needed to deal with any trouble arising from damage to the internal organs.

The outlook depends upon which parts of the body are affected. Most people manage reasonably well, but a small number succumb to kidney failure or other problems that arise when a key part of the body becomes too dry.

Polymyalgia rheumatica — the pain of many muscles

No one knows what causes *polymyalgia rheumatica,* which means *pain in many muscles.* It typically attacks people over the age of 50 and more women than men. The older you are, the more likely you are to wake up one morning with the muscle pain and stiffness that are the hallmarks of this disease.

Typically, a woman goes to bed at night feeling fine. But she wakes up the next morning with tremendous pain and stiffness in her neck, shoulders, upper arms, lower back, hips, and/or buttocks. She may say, "It feels like I worked out too much yesterday, like I really overdid it — but I didn't do anything!"

Not everyone develops polymyalgia rheumatica overnight. Sometimes it comes on gradually. In addition to the pain and stiffness, there may be fever, weight loss, and a general feeling of the "blahs."

Although the pain can be severe and may seem to resemble that of rheumatoid arthritis, the muscles involved don't show signs of inflammation, and the joints rarely show any signs of arthritis. There may, however, be inflammation of the joint linings.

With no characteristic joint damage, antibodies, skin rashes, or other obvious signs to look for, doctors must make the diagnosis of polymyalgia rheumatica by eliminating other causes of the pain and stiffness. The patient's age is one clue. Then there's the typically sudden onset of symptoms. People with the disease may also have anemia and a high erythrocyte sedimentation rate (ESR), but these are not definitive clues because they can be the result of many other health problems.

Sometimes the diagnosis is clinched by the patient's response to the standard treatment: low doses of prednisone or other corticosteroids. Almost all polymyalgia rheumatica patients respond well to low doses of these drugs.

This "pain of many muscles" often disappears on its own or improves dramatically with treatment. A significant number of patients do so well after a couple years that they can start cutting back on their medication.

Paget's disease — becoming too bony

Bones grow throughout life. They may not grow longer after a certain point, but they are constantly being broken down and restored, right up until the end of life.

With Paget's disease, the normal break down/rebuild system shifts into overdrive, causing excessive destruction of the bone and poor quality bone repair. As a result, bones may become bulkier, softer, and weaker, with a greater tendency to fracture.

Many people with Paget's have no idea anything is wrong, while others suffer from gradual joint stiffness and fatigue. Sometimes the bones become enlarged, deformed, and painful. And there can be "secondary" damage, such as pain, osteoarthritis, loss of height, and bowleggedness.

It's also possible, though not very likely, for the abnormal bone growth to stress the heart, leading to heart failure.

Making the diagnosis of Paget's is fairly simple: X rays of the bones show the abnormal areas of growth, and a laboratory test detects elevated blood levels of alkaline phosphatase, an enzyme necessary for bone formation.

Treatment depends upon the symptoms — if there are none, perhaps nothing will be done. Surgery may be needed if nerves are being pinched or if a joint is no longer functioning properly. In more severe cases, your doctor may prescribe drugs that slow the disease, such as etidronate and calcitonin, or drugs used to strengthen bones, such as alendronate sodium.

Arthritis As a Companion Condition

In these conditions, arthritis may be present, but it's a separate disease process.

Carpal tunnel syndrome: nerve compression

You may have seen office workers or supermarket checkers wearing splints on their hands and lower arms to immobilize their wrists. Or perhaps you've noticed people rubbing and shaking their hands, complaining of pain and tingling in their thumbs and fingers.

They may be suffering from carpal tunnel syndrome, a problem caused by compression of the nerve and tendons that pass through the *carpal tunnel,* a corridor between the ligaments and bones in the wrist. This causes decreased sensations, pain, numbness, and tingling in the thumb, index, and middle fingers that can sometimes spread all the way up to the arm and shoulder. If left untreated, carpal tunnel syndrome can cause the muscles on the thumb side of the hand to waste away, making it difficult to make a fist or grasp objects.

Your doctor will base the diagnosis on your symptoms, medical history, and physical examination. She or he will look for weakness and decreased sensation in the hand. An X ray may provide helpful information, and nerve tests can confirm the diagnosis.

Treatment often begins with a splint, followed by medication to reduce pain and inflammation. Corticosteroid injections into the afflicted nerve can be temporarily helpful. If the problem is related to water gain, you may be given diuretics to help get rid of excess fluid. More advanced cases may by helped by surgery.

In addition to these medical measures, look for ways to cut back on — or completely eliminate — any repetitive motion that may bring on the pain. Also, look for ways to relieve joint stress. For example, if you type a lot, consider getting an ergonomically designed keyboard.

The outlook for those with carpal tunnel syndrome is generally good. Most recover, and only a very small percentage of those treated develop permanent nerve injury.

Fibromyalgia: The pain no one can find

It's an odd situation: You hurt, perhaps all over, but the doctor can't find any inflammation or damage to explain the pain. He may even suggest "it's all in your head," that you're stressed, depressed, or that you need more sleep.

Pain and stiffness in the muscles, ligaments, and tendons are the primary signs of fibromyalgia. The pain and stiffness are generally body-wide, although they can begin in one area and spread. Fatigue is also a major problem; as many as 90 percent of fibromyalgia sufferers also experience moderate to severe fatigue.

Symptoms may come and go, and are often associated with sleep disturbances, and there may also be mood changes, numbness and tingling in the extremities, and headaches. No one knows what causes the disorder, but it is often triggered by stress, injury, lack of sleep, infections, and other diseases. Although fibromyalgia can be painful, it is not life-threatening or otherwise dangerous. For some people, however, the symptoms can be so severe that work is impossible.

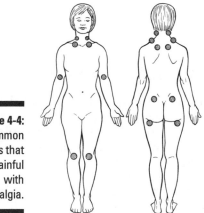

Figure 4-4:
Common areas that are painful with fibromyalgia.

The Arthritis Foundation estimates that 3.7 million Americans suffer from fibromyalgia. Women are seven times more likely than men to suffer from this condition, especially those in their childbearing years.

The diagnosis can be difficult to make, because the symptoms of fibromyalgia may be similar to those of other diseases. The location and pattern of your pain will help your doctor make the diagnosis.

Treatment may include medicines to kill pain, local anesthetics injected directly into painful areas, and antidepressants to aid in sleep. Your doctor may also prescribe exercise and application of heat and massage. Relaxation techniques and education to help you manage your pain may also be prescribed.

Fibromyalgia is not all in your head; it's not a hysterical response to stress or a cry for help. It's a real disease that happens to have an important psychological component. That's good news, in a sense, because it means you can begin doing something, right now, to help relieve your symptoms by controlling stress. (See Chapter 13 for methods of dealing with stress.) For more immediate relief, try taking a warm bath or applying compresses to your sore muscles. And you may have a little more luck sleeping with a different mattress, a "white noise" machine to block disturbing sounds, blackout curtains, and a more comfortable pillow. (See Chapter 14 for the basics of good sleep.)

Overall, the outlook for fibromyalgia patients is good. It causes no long-term damage to the joints or the rest of the body and can be eased with medicine and stress reduction.

Polymyositis — a rare sapping of strength

An uncommon disease affecting less than one tenth of one percent of the population, polymyositis is an inflammation of the muscles that saps the victim's strength. In severe cases, those with polymyositis may have trouble just lifting themselves out of a chair or brushing their teeth. It's usually the larger muscles closest to the torso that suffer — the muscles of the shoulders, upper arms, thighs, and hips. But the neck muscles may also be stricken, as well as those used to breathe and swallow. There can also be pain in the joints, fever, weight loss, Raynaud's phenomenon, and the "blahs."

Polymyositis can strike at any age, but usually hits adults between 30 and 60, and children aged 5 to 15. And the disease prefers women to men, striking the fair sex about twice as often. No one knows what causes polymyositis. Infections and immune system disorders are suspected, whereas genetics are not.

Lacking a quick and easy test that can provide a definitive diagnosis, doctors look for identifying signs and symptoms. These include unexplained muscle weakness, certain microscopic changes in the structure of the muscle tissue, and changes in the levels of certain enzymes in the blood.

A corticosteroid called prednisone, given to strengthen the muscles and quell the inflammation, is a standard medication for this disease. Unfortunately, while some people respond quickly and dramatically to this medicine, others do not. Ironically, prednisone can cause muscle *weakness* and a host of other unpleasant side effects.

Although many children stricken with the disease can stop their medication after a year or so, most adult patients continue taking their drugs for many years — or indefinitely. Some adults suffer from progressively more severe symptoms, and eventually die from respiratory failure, pneumonia, or other problems; but most are able to keep the disease under control and live fairly normal lives.

Dermatomyositis — polymyositis plus

With dermatomyositis, one suffers of all the symptoms of polymyositis, plus rashes and skin problems.

There may be a reddish rash on the face, reddish-purple swelling about the eyes, and a rash elsewhere on the body. Typically appearing on the knuckles, the rash may be raised, smooth, or scaly. With time the rash fades, but may leave behind areas with brownish pigmentation or no pigmentation at all, as well as scarred or shriveled skin.

Treatment for dermatomyositis is similar to that of polymyositis.

True Patient Stories

Many millions of people have been struck by symptoms ranging from joint stiffness to skin rashes to difficulty swallowing. Sometimes the diagnosis is made quickly. Other times, people are forced to endure myriad tests and bounce from doctor to doctor until they find out what's wrong. And along the path to diagnosis, they're often mistakenly told that their problems are caused by stress, lack of sleep, or depression. Even when the disease is identified, the course may not be clear. Many patients spend money for one medicine after another or self-refer themselves to specialists outside their managed care or HMO programs, paying for the doctors themselves in the quest for relief. Here are the experiences of some people just like you:

Recurring chest pain sent a frightened 25-year-old Kristen to her doctor.

Stricken by severe pain on the right side of his "belly" that suggested appendicitis, Franklin found himself in the hospital, about to undergo exploratory surgery.

Middle-aged Janice has felt weak and tired for the past several weeks.

After drinking too much at a New Year's party, Rod woke early in the morning with excruciating pain in his big toe.

Terry's fingers had a tendency to turn white, blue, then red; they tingled, burned, and became numb.

Fever, abdominal and joint pain sent 27 year-old Jennifer to her doctor's office.

What do these people, with such different and wide-ranging symptoms, have in common? They all have arthritis or an arthritis-related condition. Their pain is not all in their heads, and it's not due to depression or psychological problems. Their symptoms are absolutely real, and they need careful care.

Part II

Tests and Treatments: What to Expect from Your Doctor

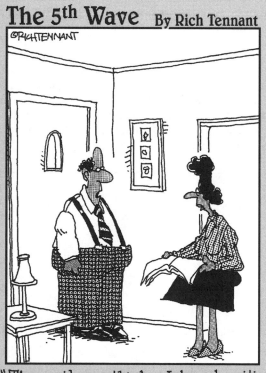

The 5th Wave   By Rich Tennant

"The mailman thinks I have bursitis, but I'd like to get a second opinion from my accountant."

In this part . . .

*1*t would be great if a single test could tell you if you had arthritis, which type, and if a single treatment is used for all the many forms of the disease. Unfortunately, such a test doesn't exist. Diagnosis can be a quick and easy or a long and drawn-out process. And making the treatment decisions can sometimes be difficult.

In this part, we explain how doctors go about diagnosing the many forms of arthritis and the high-tech and low-tech tests they may use. We also discuss the medicines they may prescribe and surgeries they may recommend. And, equally important, we show you how to work with your doctor to make treatment decisions, then how to manage any pain you may suffer.

Chapter 5

Your Doctor and You: Allies Against Arthritis

*I*n the old days — well, just 15 or 20 years ago — the doctor said, "Jump" and the patient answered, "How high?" In other words, the doctor was completely in charge, ordering tests as he or she saw fit, deciding how aggressively or conservatively to attack the disease, pushing patients toward surgery or drugs, taking a dim view of alternative approaches, and so on.

Fortunately, there's a new approach to health care today: Doctor and patient work together as a team with you, the patient, in charge. Research has shown that patients who play active roles in their treatment tend to fare better. That's why selecting your doctor carefully, helping draw up the treatment program, and then following that program to the letter is important. Your odds of recovery improve if you believe in your treatment and pitch in with your recovery efforts, doing everything you can to get well.

Don't Self-Diagnose

It can be tempting to read the descriptions of various diseases, pick out the one whose symptoms most closely match yours, and make your own diagnosis.

Some people may make the right diagnosis. But a lot of people will make the wrong diagnosis, because the symptoms of many forms of arthritis overlap with those of other forms of the disease — they can even be confused with entirely different ailments. Making the wrong diagnosis can lead to the wrong treatment, which can be dangerous.

Do not self-diagnose. No matter how obvious the situation seems, it is vital that you go to a medical doctor, have a complete examination, and get an "official" diagnosis.

The Goals of Treatment

Doctors are experts, trained well in diagnosis and treatment. They'd better be, because we put our health (and our lives) into their hands. Still, doctors are only human, which makes them subject to limitations and foibles just like the rest of us. Therefore, it's important for you to follow the three cardinal rules of treatment:

- **Select your doctor carefully.** Find someone who is not only thoroughly familiar with and experienced in treating your kind of arthritis, but is also up on the latest research and treatments. You don't want to miss out on an effective therapy because your doctor is uninformed.

- **Learn all you can about your condition.** How can you gauge whether your doctor is following correct procedure and doing all that's possible to treat your condition unless you know something about the topic? Plenty of information about every type of arthritis, its symptoms, treatments, alternative healing methods, and so on is available from the Arthritis Foundation 800-283-7800, www.arthritis.org, or similar organizations. (See Appendix B for more information.)

- **Be a team player with your doctor.** Once you've decided on a doctor, regard him or her as the expert — your trusted advisor. Unless something feels wrong about the advice you're getting, follow it to the letter. Get behind your treatment and do all you can to make it successful. Only then can you get the best possible results.

Choosing a Good Doctor

How do you find a good doctor? Ideally, you begin by getting recommendations from your friends, doctors, or other people in the medical field, your own general practitioner or internist (if you're searching for a specialist), or perhaps a highly-regarded nearby hospital or medical center. You then need to check the candidates' credentials on the Internet or call the local chapter of the American Medical Association to narrow the field. Finally, you person-ally interview those left on your now shorter list and select the doctor who seems to suit you best. However, in real life, you may not have the opportu-nity to select your doctors quite so freely — you may be restricted to the ones on the list that your insurance company or HMO provides.

Luckily, it's quite likely that you can find an excellent doctor through your HMO or on your insurance-approved list. After all, the overwhelming majority of doctors are well qualified to help. But some are undoubtedly a better match for you than others. Assuming that you have some choice, looking around for the physician best suited to your needs is worth your while. Here are three questions to ask yourself as you narrow your search:

- Is the doctor knowledgeable?
- Can the two of you work together?
- Do you share the same philosophy?

Is the doctor knowledgeable?

Almost every doctor has an office wall full of diplomas and certificates, and although you may find them interesting to look at, most of these fancy, framed pieces of paper can't offer you much useful information. Not even a diploma from Harvard Medical School, you ask? Isn't a diploma from a super-prestigious school better than one from Tiny Town Med? Not necessarily. Plenty of brilliant doctors have graduated from little-known medical colleges.

What about the official-looking paper that the state issues proclaiming that the doctor is licensed to practice medicine? Remember that every practicing physician *has* to have one of those to treat patients. (It's like a driver's license for doctors.)

As for membership in the American Medical Association, the AMA is primar-ily a trade association. If Dr. Smith can pay the dues, he can join the AMA, but that doesn't necessarily mean he's better than a non-AMA doctor.

And what about the certificates indicating that the doctor is a member of var-ious medical societies? Again, these documents guarantee nothing. A doctor can belong to an organization that offers wonderful seminars and educational materials, yet never once take advantage of them. On the other hand, a doctor who doesn't belong to a medical organization may spend hours study-ing medical journals and swapping tips with colleagues. What if the doctor is a diplomate in a medical society? Sometimes this title can mean something. Certain medical societies require that their members pass rigorous written tests before allowing the doctors to call themselves diplomates. On the other hand, some societies offer diplomate tests that aren't so difficult.

The one thing that *does* mean something is board certification. *Board-certified* means that the doctor has passed difficult written and/or oral tests in his or her field. Certification is generally considered an impressive credential, because it isn't required to practice. Being board-certified is an extra stamp of validation that not every doctor receives.

Can the two of you work together?

Once you're sure that your prospective physician is qualified, you must try to predict whether the two of you can work together. Don't automatically assume that the answer is yes. You, the patient, should be considered a member of the treatment team — the most important member — rather than a passive pin cushion who acquiesces to whatever medicines and/or surgeries your doctor deems necessary. How can you find out if your prospective doctor seems like a team player?

After you visit with a doctor for either an interview or an appointment, think carefully about what went on during your time together. Did he or she:

- ✔ Try to rush you through the interview?

- ✔ Keep looking at his or her watch?

- ✔ Solicit your opinions?

- ✔ Give you ample time to express your thoughts, wishes, concerns, and fears?

- ✔ Listen carefully?

- ✔ Give you thoughtful, complete responses in plain English (instead of confusing medical speak)?

- ✔ Invite you to ask questions?

- ✔ Ask about your preferred approach to treatment? (For example, whether you'd like to begin treatment with strong painkillers or if you prefer to give exercise and a back brace a chance before moving on to medication?)

- ✔ Push you to pursue much more aggressive or conservative treatment than you prefer?

- ✔ Brush aside your concerns by saying, "Trust me" or "I know what's best?"

- ✔ Focus on drugs and/or surgery for treatment and downplay your desire to work with a physical therapist, chiropractor, or other alternative healer?

There are no correct answers to any of these questions, and you can't rank the doctor on the "He's For Me" scale. However, you can learn a lot by asking questions, listening carefully, and observing the doctor's behavior.

Do you share the same treatment philosophy?

Many people think of medicine as a science, but it's often just as much an art. For example, doctors frequently follow hunches during their diagnostic workup. And although there are standard approaches to treating most diseases, doctors know that everybody responds a little differently. Therefore, most treatment programs must be individualized, and then changed as time goes on — anywhere from slightly tweaked to altered radically.

Because everyone responds to treatment differently, physicians have some leeway when diagnosing and treating patients — some wiggle room that also allows for the expression of personality. Some doctors are more aggressive than others; some like the idea of alternative approaches, while others are determined to stick strictly to Western medical techniques. Some doctors want to tell you exactly what to do, while others are more willing to involve you in the decision-making process.

Although no diploma hanging on the wall is going to let you in on a doctor's treatment philosophy, it may offer you some clues. Framed certificates of membership in medical or non-medical organizations dedicated to nutrition or exercise, for example, or certificates stating that the doctor has attended lectures in chiropractic or herbal medicine suggest that the doctor is open to alternative therapies. But the best way, by far, to learn about a doctor's philosophy about diagnosis and treatment is simply to ask. You may find the following questions helpful:

- ✔ Do you consider yourself aggressive or conservative in treating disease?
- ✔ Do you think medication is always, or almost always, the best treatment for arthritis?
- ✔ How valuable are diet, exercise, and stress reduction in treating arthritis?
- ✔ Do you favor the use of vitamins, herbs, and other supplements as adjuncts to treatment? If so, which ones?
- ✔ How do you feel about using other alternative therapies (chiropractic, massage, homeopathy, magnets, acupuncture, and so on) in conjunction with standard treatment? Which do you feel are best?

There are no right answers to these questions. Ideally, you'll find that the doctor's attitudes toward treatment dovetail with yours.

General practitioner versus rheumatologist

Whether you need a specialist depends upon the kind of arthritis you have. If you have osteoarthritis, you may do well under the care of a general practitioner or internist. But if you have a more complicated kind of arthritis, one that involves entire body systems (such as rheumatoid arthritis), you'll probably need to see a *rheumatologist*.

Rheumatologists specialize in diseases of the joints, muscles, and bones and treat arthritis, musculoskeletal pain disorders, osteoporosis, and various autoimmune diseases. An important part of the rheumatologist's job is proper diagnosis of the disease, because symptoms can point to many different conditions. After the rheumatologist pinpoints the disease, proper treatment can begin, so early and accurate diagnosis is crucial. If you don't have a clear-cut case of osteoarthritis, or if your family physician or internist seems baffled by your symptoms, consult a rheumatologist.

Talking with Your Doctor

Although you're not expected to know everything (any more than an orchestra conductor has to play every instrument proficiently), you do need to know enough to communicate with your doctor(s) and the other members of your medical team. Doing so requires a certain amount of education. You needn't become an expert, and you don't have to stay up all night mastering arcane medical terms and memorizing medical books. However, you should read and learn all you can about the type of arthritis you have, as well as the medications that have been prescribed, to become conversant about your disease. Some good information sources include the following:

- ✔ ***The Merck Manual of Medical Information, Home Edition.*** This is the layman's version of the technical manual that doctors use.

- ✔ ***The PDR Pocket Guide to Prescription Drugs.*** This is a slimmed-down and simplified version of the *PDR (Physician's Desk Reference),* the doctor's reference guide to medications. In regular, non-doctor English, *The PDR Pocket Guide* spells out important issues concerning each medication, such as:

  - Why it's prescribed

  - The most important facts about the drug

  - Tips on how you should take the medication

  - Side effects

  - Tips for when you shouldn't use the drug

  - Clues concerning how the drug may interact with foods and other drugs

✔ **Arthritis support groups.** Consider joining an arthritis support group. The other members understand what you're going through, so they'll listen sympathetically, and they've been in your situation, so they can give you helpful advice. Likewise, if you join the group, at some point you'll become a regular, which gives you the great satisfaction of helping others. You can find support groups by asking your doctor, nurses, or the community support staff at your hospital.

You can also find arthritis support groups through the Arthritis Foundation. Give them a call at 800-283-7800 or check out their Web site at www.arthritis.org. If you go to their Web site, click "Arthritis Answers," then scroll down and click "Local Offices" in the left-hand column to find the Arthritis Foundation office nearest you. Give them a call to ask for the location and meeting time of a support group in your area.

✔ **The Internet.** Three great places to begin your search are the Arthritis Foundation (www.arthritis.org), the National Institute of Arthritis and Musculoskeletal and Skin Diseases (www.nih.gov/niams) and the American College of Rheumatology (www.rheumatology.org). You can also find more Web sites in Appendix B of this book.

The Internet is a great place to learn. Unfortunately, you can't treat everything you find there as the gospel. Before accepting what you read, ask yourself who is offering the material, who wrote the material, why it was written, and when. If the information is offered by well-known, reputable organizations, such as the Arthritis Foundation, the National Institute of Arthritis and Musculoskeletal Diseases, or the American College of Rheumatology, it's undoubtedly good information. However, if an organization devoted to selling products mentioned in the literature prepares and posts the information you find, take what you read with a grain of salt.

No matter where you find information, ask yourself who wrote it: A physician or other health professional? A respected non-medical educator? Some guy off the street? Is the author qualified to present information or give advice? Ask yourself if the article is offered as information or if it's designed to sell a product. There's nothing wrong with selling products, and some pieces that are written with the idea of selling are packed with unbiased, useful information. However, others aren't. Be sure to check the date that the information was posted. Even a well-researched article may contain erroneous information if it hasn't been updated in several years.

When Should You Find a New Doctor?

Not every marriage is made in heaven, and not every patient/doctor partnership works out for the best. If you're wondering whether it's time to switch to a different doctor, ask yourself the following questions, adapted from the article "Red Flags" by Doyt Conn, M.D.:

✔ **Do you feel the progress of your treatment is too slow?** It may take awhile before your doctor finds the right treatment for you, and complete relief of your symptoms isn't always possible. If your doctor is still trying to adjust your treatment, you may want to stick it out a little longer. If not, find someone else.

✔ **Does your treatment consist of medication only?** Treatment of arthritis is multifaceted and should include nondrug therapies often, such as exercise, diet, joint protection techniques, rest, and so on.

✔ **Does your doctor rely on NSAIDs?** NSAIDs were once the treatment-of-choice for arthritis. But acetaminophen may be a better choice for you if you have osteoarthritis, because NSAIDs are notorious for causing stomach problems. Also, treatment of rheumatoid arthritis may require the use of more aggressive drugs (such as methotrexate or sulfasalazine). In some cases, delaying the use of these drugs may cause the affected joints to become irreparably damaged.

✔ **Does your doctor regularly give you cortisone injections for flares?** Although injecting cortisone into an inflamed joint is a fast way of stopping an RA flare, doing so on a regular basis can lay the groundwork for an even worse flare after the medication wears off. Doctors who rely on this method can end up doing more harm than good.

Generally, the best advice is to go with your gut feeling. If something feels wrong or you and your doctor don't seem to click, find someone with whom you do feel comfortable. Having confidence in the type and quality of medical care that you receive can make a positive difference in your recovery.

Chapter 6

Judging Joint Health with Low- and High-Tech Tests

In This Chapter

▶ Learning what a good doctor does to diagnose arthritis

▶ Introducing common tests for the various forms of arthritis

▶ Finding out which tests are used to help pin down your diagnosis

iagnosing arthritis can be as easy as 1-2-3. Or it may take months or even years of following up on clues and running endless tests. With osteoarthritis, the diagnosis is usually pretty clear: the patient is typically over 40, has pain but no swelling in a singular joint, and an X ray shows ragged or worn cartilage. But with other forms of arthritis, such as Lyme disease, the symptoms can be much more vague: fatigue, chills, fever, rash, inflammation of the heart, meningitis, and joint aches that may come and go for years. However, doctors have many tests available to narrow the long list of possibilities and pinpoint a diagnosis.

Medical History and Physical Exam

There's no one test that can tell for sure whether or not you have arthritis. Instead, your doctor will go through several procedures, such as taking a thorough medical history, examining you carefully, and performing a series of tests. Together, these "clues" should provide a pretty accurate picture of what's going on in your body.

Medical history

Your doctor will want to assemble a great deal of information about your overall health, as well as your specific complaints. The medical history should include general information such as your age, sex, and occupation.

It should also include specific information about any accidents or injuries that you've sustained and diseases that run in your family. Your doctor needs to know about any illnesses you've had (especially recently) and any other problems, including recent weight loss, depression, sleep disturbances, aches and pain, skin changes, and fatigue.

The doctor should also review your activities at work and home and those you do for leisure. Knowing that you type eight hours a day may help the doctor connect your hand pain and tingling to carpal tunnel syndrome, while knowing that you drink a lot of alcohol may point to the possibility of gout. You might help guide your doctor to the diagnosis of Lyme disease by revealing that you went camping in the woods and discovered a rash on your back shortly before your joints began hurting. And, of course, you should tell the doctor about any and all of your symptoms.

Don't hold back information because you think it's not important. You may not mention that you've had some difficulty in swallowing because you don't think it's related to your joint and muscle pain. But if you have scleroderma or polymyositis, it very well may be.

The physical exam

Even if you only have pain in a single joint, you should be examined from head to toe. Your primary physician (internist or family practitioner is the most likely one to do this. If you see a rheumatologist or other specialist, he or she probably won't look you over from stem to stern but should carefully examine all affected and related areas.

How important is the head-to-toe examination? Well, urinary difficulties in men can be due to Reiter's Syndrome, gonococcal arthritis, or something totally different, such as an enlarged prostate gland. Without a thorough examination, the proper diagnosis may be missed.

At some point, the examination will focus on your painful joint(s). Your doctor will be particularly interested in the following key symptoms:

- ✔ How many joints are affected?
- ✔ Does the pain affect the same joints on both sides of the body?
- ✔ Does redness, swelling, and warmth surround the joint, and is it tender to the touch?

The doctor will ask you to bend and straighten your affected joint(s) several times as he determines the range of motion. He will manipulate your joints(s) for you, checking for joint crackling and pain upon bending and flexing. Your doctor will also examine any related areas and check your reflexes and muscle strength.

Arthritis timeline

200,000,000 BC: A dinosaur roared in pain when struck by osteoarthritis. We know this is true because examination of dinosaur bones shows evidence of the disease.

2,000,000 BC: An otherwise unknown ape-man developed chronic arthritis of the spine. He may not have been the first human to do so, but he's the oldest of those whose arthritic bones have been found.

8,000 BC: An Egyptian important enough to be mummified had the evidence of his arthritis wrapped up with him.

440 BC: Hippocrates, the father of Western medicine, offered the first known description of arthritis. He described gout as a "violent attack on the joints."

Circa 300 AD: Arthritis was so endemic in the Roman Empire that the Emperor Diocletian gave a tax break to the citizens who were most afflicted with the disease.

Circa 400 AD: Colchicum, from which the drug colchicine is derived today, was introduced as a treatment for gout.

Circa 1600 AD: Guilaurne de Bailou introduced the term *rheumatism* and suggested that it was a type of arthritis different from gout.

1907 AD: X rays were added to doctors' diagnostic arsenal, allowing them to further distinguish one type of arthritis from another.

1949: The rheumatoid factor, which plays a role in rheumatoid arthritis, was discovered. In the same year, cortisone was introduced as a treatment for this disease.

1951 AD: Drugs to suppress an errant immune system and modify the course of rheumatoid arthritis were first used.

1960 AD: Surgeons began performing total joint replacement.

Early 1960s AD: The urate crystals that cause gout were identified, and new drugs to control the disease were introduced.

1963 AD: New NSAIDs (non-steroidal anti-inflammatory drugs), useful in controlling arthritic inflammation, were introduced.

1977 AD: Lyme disease was recognized and named.

The doctor may ask you to walk, sit, rise from a chair, bend, and do other movements so he or she can assess the way you use your joints. You may be asked to reach for something or make a fist around a pencil so the doctor can estimate the impact of your condition on your ability to perform daily activities.

Assessing the pain and other symptoms

You and your doctor will discuss in detail the kind and amount of pain you're experiencing, and you will need to answer questions that are specifically geared to the pain itself. You may want to pay special attention to these issues before you see your doctor so that you can have your answers ready. The following is a Pain Checklist for you to check off symptoms, write in your own comments, and take with you to your doctor's appointment.

❑ Is it an ache, a burn, a throb, or a stabbing pain?

❑ Does it come and go, or is it constant?

❑ What activities or movements make the pain worse?

❑ What makes the pain recede?

❑ Are you stiff in the morning?

❑ Do your joints lock up?

❑ Is the pain more intense at a certain time of day?

❑ How does your condition affect your work and home life?

You may also be asked to rate your pain on a scale of 1 to 10, with 10 being intolerable pain.

If you keep a "pain diary" or "symptom diary" for several days or weeks before visiting your doctor, you'll be able to paint a more accurate picture of your pain and other problems.

X Rays, Scans, and Biopsies

Usually, an X ray is the one of the first diagnostic tools that doctors order for patients. X rays are useful in diagnosing and distinguishing between two of the most common forms of arthritis: osteoarthritis and rheumatoid arthritis.

Other forms of arthritis must be diagnosed with other tools available, including scans and biopsies. You may have just an X ray, or an MRI plus a biopsy; it all depends on what your doctor deems necessary.

Ordering an X ray

X rays are particularly helpful in confirming that cartilage and/or joint damage does exist and in distinguishing between osteoarthritis and rheumatoid arthritis. Ankylosing spondylitis and similar conditions can also be confirmed with an X ray.

In osteoarthritis, roughened bone ends, cartilage deterioration, uneven narrowing of the joint space, bone spurs, and thickened bone ends can be seen clearly in an X ray. A joint afflicted with RA will show tissue swelling, decreased bone density, narrowing of the joint space in an even manner, and possibly bone erosion. In ankylosing spondylitis, X rays can reveal inflammation, small bone growths, and other changes in the sacroiliac joints.

X rays are very helpful in detecting rheumatoid arthritis, osteoarthritis, and Reiter's syndrome, but aren't so useful in diagnosing gout, Raynaud's phenomenon, or bursitis.

Scans

Sometimes a standard X ray can't tell the doctor what he or she needs to know, because they can't produce images of soft tissue or give the doctor a three-dimensional view. That's where CAT scans and MRIs come in handy.

- **MRI scans:** MRI stands for magnetic resonance imaging (MRI). Magnetism, radio waves, and a computer are used to create detailed images of body structures. MRIs are especially helpful in diagnosing lupus, ankylosing spondylitis, and other ailments that affect soft tissues. You'll lie on a table as the scan is taken. It used to be that the patient was placed on a table inside a tunnel made of scanning machinery during the MRI. Today, there are *open MRIs* in which you don't feel so claustrophobic.

- **CAT scans:** The CAT scan (which stands for computerized axial tomography) is a marriage of X rays and computer technology in which a series of X rays of one area are taken from different angles. The computer builds these images into three-dimensional pictures. This can be helpful in diagnosing, for example, lupus, problems with the spine and soft tissues. For a CAT scan, you'll lie on narrow table inside a tunnel-like scanner. The bad part is that the scan takes an average of an hour and a half, you can feel claustrophobic lying in the tunnel, and the machine makes a great deal of noise.

Biopsies

Samples of the skin, muscle, kidneys, liver, arteries, or nerves may be taken to confirm diagnoses of the more unusual types of arthritis. For example, a muscle biopsy can help in the diagnosis of polymyositis; a skin biopsy may be necessary to corroborate psoriatic arthritis, lupus, or scleroderma; while a biopsy of joint fluid can help make the diagnosis of gout, pseudogout, infectious arthritis, or Reiter's Syndrome.

Testing the Blood

Blood tests can help confirm a tentative diagnosis or rule out other causes of joint pain. Certain substances found in the blood can indicate inflammation, infections, muscle damage, or other signs of a particular type of arthritis. For example, the presence of RA factor suggests rheumatoid arthritis; certain antibody abnormalities can suggest lupus; while the presence of antibodies to *Borrelia burgdorferi* indicate Lyme disease. Common blood tests for the various kinds of arthritis include:

✔ **Anti-DNA and Anti-Sm:** Antibodies to DNA, the cell's genetic material, and Sm, another substance found in the nucleus of the cell, are commonly found in those with lupus.

Because these antibodies are rarely present in the blood of people who don't have lupus, this test is a reliable diagnostic tool.

✔ **Blood chemistries:** Abnormal amounts of various chemical substances can indicate the possibility of certain forms of arthritis. A high level of uric acid, for example, can be a sign of gout. High levels of creatinine kinase indicate disturbed kidney function, which may indicate lupus or another disease of the connective tissue. A positive result obtained from the Lyme serology blood tests means that antibodies have been produced to fight an organism transmitted through a tick bite.

However, blood abnormalities can often point to many different diseases, so these tests are usually used to supply diagnostic clues only.

✔ **Complement:** A group of blood proteins that are activated as part of the immune process, the complement system releases substances that kill bacteria and send white blood cells rushing to fight off invaders. A low complement level suggests that your immune system is working in overdrive and that you may have a disease, perhaps lupus.

✔ **Complete Blood Count (CBC):** While the presence of arthritis can't be confirmed by a CBC, it can be indicated. For example, a low red blood cell count (anemia) can be a sign of chronic inflammation, which is found in rheumatoid arthritis, Sjögren's Syndrome, or polymyalgia rheumatica. A high white cell count may signal some kind of infectious arthritis, such as Lyme disease, Reiter's syndrome, or gonococcal arthritis. Low levels of blood platelets may be another indication of rheumatoid arthritis.

✔ **Erythrocyte sedimentation rate (ESR):** During inflammation, the red blood cells (*erythrocytes*) clump together, becoming heavier than normal. When left to stand in a test tube, these heavy red blood cells will fall faster than normal. The rate at which your red blood cells settle in a one-hour period is called the *erythrocyte sedimentation rate* or *ESR*. A high ESR indicates inflammation.

✔ **Fluorescent antinuclear antibody (FANA):** More than 95 percent of lupus patients have antibodies that attack and take over the nuclei of healthy cells (*antinuclear antibodies*). The fluorescent dye used in the FANA test can show these antibodies clinging to the cell nuclei. Because this test requires the utmost skill in the laboratory to ensure correct results, it may have to be repeated. Besides those with lupus, up to 50 percent of patients with RA and even some healthy patients register as positive on the FANA test.

✔ **Rheumatoid factor (RF):** About 80 percent of patients with rheumatoid arthritis have an antibody called *rheumatoid factor (RF)* in their blood. No one is quite sure whether RF causes the disease or is the result of the immune system's reaction to the disease. Although it's a pretty good indicator of rheumatoid arthritis, some people with RA don't have the factor, and some who do have the factor don't have RA. Like most blood tests, this one must be factored in with other symptoms before an accurate diagnosis can be made.

These are not the only blood tests that your doctor may order, and the examples given are not the only reasons for using them. They are, however, common among the tests doctors use.

Other Tests to Make the Diagnosis

Doctors have a good idea of what may be wrong after listening to you describe your symptoms, examining you, and considering your medical history. With many forms of arthritis, they may need nothing more than an X ray or scan, a blood test and/or a biopsy to confirm the diagnosis. However, sometimes more testing is necessary. If, for example, gout is suspected, a sample of joint fluid may need to be drawn and examined in the laboratory. If ankylosing spondylitis is likely, genetic testing may be required. Here are some "other" tests:

Examining the joint fluid

Your doctor may want to insert a needle into one or all of your affected joints to withdraw a small amount of fluid for examination under a microscope. He or she can draw out additional fluid to help relieve pain and pressure inside of your joint, if the swelling is intense.

Called *joint aspiration* or *tapping a joint,* the doctor sterilizes the area, uses a local anesthetic, inserts a needle then pulls out a small amount of fluid (as little as a couple of drops or as much as a tablespoon or two). He or she then sends the joint fluid to a laboratory for analysis.

Healthy joints contain clear fluid; anything else is probably an indication of a problem. Blood in the fluid may be the result of a substantial injury to the joint. Cloudy fluid or the presence of large numbers of white blood cells (pus) is an indication of either infectious or inflammatory arthritis. Crystals in the fluid are probably due to gout or pseudogout. Bits of cartilage or bone present in otherwise clear fluid usually indicate osteoarthritis.

Arthroscopy

An arthroscope (a fiberoptic camera that's about as big around as a straw) is inserted into your joint through a small incision, allowing the doctor to check out your joint's insides in all their glory. The doctor may use this as a diagnostic tool or even as a way to perform surgery inside your joint, repairing torn cartilage, cutting away inflamed or diseased tissues, removing bits of bone or cartilage, and/or reconstructing ligaments. Only orthopedic surgeons perform arthroscopy.

Genetic Testing

Scientists have discovered that certain genes may be associated with certain types of arthritis. The genetic marker HLA-B27, for example, is often found in those with ankylosing spondylitis. HLA-DR4 (known as the rheumatoid factor) occurs in 80 percent of adults with RA. Doctors cannot rely soley on genetic testing because many people who have these genes do not get arthritis, and many who do have arthritis don't have these genes. But these tests may show an inclination toward developing a particular kind of arthritis.

Urine test

If your urine contains protein, red blood cells, or other abnormal substances, it could be an indication of kidney damage. Damage to the kidneys can be a symptom of lupus or other ailments.

Chapter 7

Medicines for Arthritis, from Aspirin to Steroids

. . . .

In This Chapter

▶ Using different classes of arthritis medications and when their use is appropriate

▶ Treating different forms of arthritis with the medications that doctors typically prescribe

▶ Figuring out the purpose of each of drug, what it does, the side effects, and other related drugs.

. . . .

Many of the medicines that doctors may prescribe for arthritis are briefly described in this chapter. Naturally, whether any of these medications may be right for you is a decision that you and your doctor should make together.

Talking to Your Doctor

It's your doctor's job to diagnose and treat, but that's an important task that can't be done without your help. To diagnose and treat your condition properly, your doctor must be thoroughly familiar with all of your symptoms — and you're the only one who can supply that information. He or she will undoubtedly ask a lot of questions to build a "knowledge database," but the doctor probably won't think of everything. If you haven't already been asked, be sure to give this information to your doctor:

✔ List everything that's bothering you. You should relate every little symptom and problem, whether physical, mental, or emotional.

✔ Tell him or her about all of your allergies and any allergic reactions you've had to any medications.

✔ List every prescription and nonprescription medicine you are taking, as well as any vitamins, minerals, amino acids, herbs, other supplements, weight loss products, muscle builders, and so on.

✔ List every medicinal cream or ointment you are using.

✔ If you are pregnant, planning to become pregnant, or are nursing, be sure to mention this to your doctor.

✔ Inform the doctor if you are on hormone replacement therapy.

✔ List the foods that you like to eat. (Grapefruit, for example, can interfere with the workings of some medicines.)

✔ Tell him what chemicals, liquids, or fumes you are exposed to at work and at home.

✔ Explain the tasks you handle at work and home, and tell him about your hobbies and recreational activities.

In short, tell your doctor all about yourself, your job, your habits, and every-thing you are ingesting. Tell him about your previous experience with medi-cines, even if it was good. (Knowing that you tolerated a certain drug well may help your doctor choose a new medicine for you or persuade him to stick with the same one.) The more your doctor knows about you, the better off you'll be. If you're not asked for the information, volunteer it.

The following questions are good ones to ask your doctor concerning any medications prescribed for you:

✔ How do I take this drug, exactly? (With or without food, in the morning, with fluid, after shaking the bottle, and so on.)

✔ What activities are safe for me to do while I'm taking this medication? (For example, can I drive? Take other medicines? Take my vitamins?)

✔ Are there any drugs, supplements, foods, or anything else that I should avoid while I'm taking this medicine?

✔ What will my pill or capsule look like? Get a picture from the PDR (*Physician's Drug Reference*), *Pocket Guide to Prescription Drugs* or a simi-lar book. Compare what the doctor or pharmacist gives you to the description or picture of the drug to make sure you have the right thing.

Doctors love to use big words, especially when talking about drugs. When you talk to your doctor, you're likely to hear him or her toss around words such as *analgesic, antimalarials, NSAIDs, immunosuppressants,* and so on. If your doctor uses *any* word that you don't understand, ask for a definition. You may also want to ask your doctor to spell it for you.

Generic equivalent, generic name, brand name: I'm so confused!

Generic name and **brand name** — The *generic name* is the medication's official moniker, bestowed upon it by the United States Adopted Names Council. The *brand name*, on the other hand, is a proprietary name given to the medication by the pharmaceutical company that owns it. Generic names often tell you something about the drug's structure or chemical formula. As far as lay people are concerned, generic names tend to be dull and unpronounceable. But brand names are often chosen with an eye toward "sales sizzle." For example, the drug with the generic name of methotrexate is sold under the brand name Rheumatrex.

You can quickly distinguish generic from brand names by looking at how they're written: generic names begin with lowercase letters, brand names start with capitals. (This doesn't work when the drug name appears at the beginning of a sentence, of course, where it will always be capitalized.)

A drug sold under its generic name is chemically equivalent to the one your doctor prescribes under its brand name. However, generic equivalent drugs don't always have the identical medicinal effect. That's why it's important to discuss generic equivalents with your doctor to make sure you're getting what you need.

It's not just gulp and swallow

Medicines are tricky. Some are best absorbed on an empty stomach, so you must be sure to take them between meals. Others can irritate the stomach, so you should take them with food. You take some long-lasting medicines once a day; others only work for a brief period of time and must be taken them several times a day. Sometimes it's necessary to have a constant level of the drug in your body, so you need to take it according to a rigid schedule. Other drugs may be taken whenever you feel they are necessary. Some medicines mix well with others, while others do not.

The point is that there's more to taking medicines than gulp and swallow. Ask your doctor for precise instructions on taking all your medicines: when, how (for example, with or without food), how often, and so on. Ask what to do if you forget to take a dose. Ask what side effects you can expect; which of them are dangerous and which are not?

If your doctor doesn't tell you all about the medicine(s), don't be afraid to ask!

The Four Classes of Drugs for Arthritis

Before deciding exactly which drug to prescribe, doctors first consider which "class" of medication is best. There are several primary classes to choose from: NSAIDs, corticosteroids, immunosupressants and DMARDs.

NSAIDs

NSAIDs (nonsteroidal anti-inflammatory drugs) help relieve pain and reduce inflammation by interfering with an enzyme called COX (cyclooxygenase). Widely used for many forms of arthritis, NSAIDs come in prescription and nonprescription (over-the-counter) variations, ranging from the familiar ibuprofen to Feldene, from Anaprox to Tolectin. The over-the-counter variations you can buy in supermarkets and drug stores have lower dosages and are generally well-tolerated. The more powerful prescription forms, on the other hand, can trigger numerous side effects, often centered in the stomach. As you'll see in the review of medicines later in this chapter, some of these side effects are potentially dangerous.

Aspirin, perhaps the best known of the NSAIDs, is available under several brand names and also as plain old aspirin. It works by interfering with the body's manufacture of the inflammation products that cause swelling, pain, and other problems. Aspirin's side effects are similar to those seen with the other NSAIDs, and it has a few more all its own.

Corticosteroids

Corticosteroids are man-made versions of certain natural hormones that your body produces. And, just like the "real thing," they can be quite powerful in both good and bad ways. The corticosteroids, including prednisone, hydrocortisone, and methylprednisolone, are powerful anti-inflammatories. Unfortunately, they have significant side effects, including increased risk of infection, elevated blood pressure, ulcers in the stomach, and thinning of the bones and skin. It's because of these side effects that doctors look for the lowest effective dose when prescribing these medicines. Corticosteroids may be used to treat rheumatoid arthritis, osteoarthritis, systemic lupus erythematosus, polymyositis, and other forms of arthritis.

Immunosuppressants

You've probably read about immunosupressants and the role they play in preventing the body from rejecting a new organ after transplant surgery. They're also used to reduce the inflammation found in some forms of arthritis. They do this by dampening the immune system's errant response. Some of these drugs prevent certain cells from growing and/or dividing, while others suppress the activity of white blood cells, major players in the immune system. Cyclophosphamide, methotrexate, and azathioprine are three well-known immunosuppressants. Side effects of the immunosuppressants include various gastrointestinal problems, low blood counts, kidney damage, and increased risk of infection and other diseases, including cancer. Rheumatoid arthritis, systemic lupus erythematosus, and ankylosing spondylitis are forms of arthritis that may call for immunosuppressives.

DMARDs

DMARDs (disease-modifying, anti-rheumatic drugs) are generally reserved for serious forms of arthritis — such as rheumatoid arthritis, psoriatic arthritis, and ankylosing spondylitis — that are not helped by other medicines. Also known as *slow-acting drugs*, *remittive drugs* or *second-line drugs*, the DMARDs apparently alter the way in which the immune system works, slowing or halting its disastrous attack on the body. Gold compounds, penicillamine, and antimalarials are some of the DMARDs.

Specific Medicines for Specific Types of Arthritis

In addition to NSAIDs, corticosteroids, immunosuppressants, and DMARDs, doctors may prescribe muscle relaxants, sleeping pills, anti-anxiety drugs, or narcotics. And, when treating some forms of arthritis and related conditions, they may prescribe drugs that deal with problems extending beyond your joints. For example, people with Raynaud's Phenomenon are often treated with drugs normally thought of as heart medications, such as *vasodilators*, to open up (dilate) the blood vessels. Unfortunately, some drugs may also be necessary to counteract or ameliorate the side effects of arthritis medicines.

No matter what medication you take, remember that you must always get complete instructions from your doctor, and follow those instructions carefully. If anything seems amiss or if you have any questions, ask your doctor!

Following is a list of some of the drugs that a doctor may prescribe for arthritis and arthritis-related conditions. In most cases, we have listed them under their brand names, with their generic names included in the discussion that follows.

Anaprox

Anaprox (generic name, naproxen sodium), also available as Naprelan and Aleve, is an NSAID used for osteoarthritis, rheumatoid arthritis, tendonitis, bursitis, gout, juvenile rheumatoid arthritis, ankylosing spondylitis, and others. It reduces joint pain, swelling, inflammation, and stiffness.

Some possible side effects include abdominal pain, diarrhea or constipation, indigestion, breathing difficulties, headache, dizziness, sweating, and fluid retention. See your doctor regularly to monitor for possible internal bleeding, ulcers, and so on.

Ansaid

Ansaid (generic name, flurbiprofen), is an NSAID used for osteoarthritis and rheumatoid arthritis. It reduces joint pain, swelling, inflammation, and stiffness.

Some possible side effects include headache, swelling, infections of the urinary tract, gastrointestinal upset, the "blahs," anxiety, and an altered sense of smell. See your doctor regularly to monitor for possible internal bleeding, ulcers, and so on.

Aspirin is an NSAID used for various types of arthritis. It reduces pain, inflammation, and fever. It's available under various names, such as Bayer, Empirin, and Ecotrin.

Some possible side effects include bleeding stomach ulcers, stomach pain, upset stomach, and heartburn. Aspirin may also cause complications during pregnancy.

Azulfidine

Azulfidine (generic name, sulfasalazine) is an anti-inflammatory and antibiotic used for rheumatoid arthritis and for ankylosing spondylitis.

Some possible side effects include bluish skin discoloration, hives, nausea, vomiting, loss of appetite, and headaches.

Ceftin

Ceftin (generic name, cefuroxime axetil) is an antibiotic used for early stage Lyme Disease.

Some possible side effects include nausea, vomiting, diarrhea, and bowel inflammation. With long-term use, bacteria that are not destroyed by Ceftin may grow in large numbers and cause a secondary infection.

Celecoxib

See Chapter 23.

Celebrex

See Chapter 23.

Cipro

Cipro (generic name, ciprofloxacin hydrochloride) is an antibiotic used for bone and joint infections.

Some possible side effects include nausea, vomiting, restlessness, headache, rash, confusion, depression, fainting, flare-up of gout symptoms, and nightmares.

Clinoril

Clinoril (generic name, sulindac) is an NSAID used for osteoarthritis, rheumatoid arthritis, bursitis, tendonitis, gout, and ankylosing spondylitis. It reduces joint pain, swelling, inflammation, and stiffness.

Some possible side effects include headache, nervousness, ringing in the ears, swelling, many stomach problems including pain, diarrhea, constipation, nausea, and loss of appetite. See your doctor regularly to monitor for possible internal bleeding, ulcers, and so on.

ColBenemid

ColBenemid (generic name, probenecid-colchicine) is a urate blocker used for acute gout. ColBenemid contains both colchicine and probenecid.

Some possible side effects include muscle weakness, nausea, vomiting, diarrhea, and blood and kidney problems. Probenecid can trigger dizziness, headaches, fever, and blood problems.

Cytoxan

Cytoxan (generic name, cyclophosphamide) is an anticancer drug used for serious cases of rheumatoid arthritis and systemic lupus erythematosus. It apparently kills some of the white blood cells that bring on the arthritis symptoms.

Some possible side effects are bleeding, pain upon urination, loss of appetite, baldness, mouth ulcers, and abdominal pain.

Daypro

Daypro (generic name, oxaprozin) is an NSAID used for osteoarthritis and rheumatoid arthritis.

Some possible side effects are rashes, depression, confusion, indigestion, nausea, and constipation. See your doctor regularly to monitor for possible internal bleeding, ulcers, and so on.

Decadron

Decadron (generic name, dexamethasone) is a corticosteroid used for rheumatoid arthritis and lupus. It reduces inflammation.

Some possible side effects are blood clots, bone problems, congestive heart failure, allergic reactions, elevated blood pressure, headaches, menstrual irregularity, peptic ulcers, and exacerbation of sugar diabetes.

This drug can increase susceptibility to infections. It can also "hide" the presence of infections.

Deltasone

Deltasone (generic name, prednisone) is a steroid used for rheumatoid arthritis and lupus. It reduces inflammation.

Some possible side effects are mood and personality changes, fluid retention, elevated blood pressure, vision problems, and exacerbation of sugar diabetes.

This drug can increase the susceptibility to infections. It can also "hide" the presence of infections.

Disalcid

Disalcid (generic name salsalate) is an NSAID used for osteoarthritis, rheumatoid arthritis, and others. It relieves pain.

Some possible side effects include nausea, rashes, ringing in the ears, and hearing problems. It contains salicylate, which has been linked to Reye's syndrome in children.

Dolobid

Dolobid (generic name, diflunisal) is an NSAID used for osteoarthritis and rheumatoid arthritis. It reduces joint pain, swelling, inflammation, and stiffness.

Some possible side effects include sleepiness, insomnia, dizziness, fatigue, headaches, ringing in the ears, abdominal pain, kidney failure, vomiting, and flatulence. See your doctor regularly to monitor for possible internal bleeding, ulcers, and so on.

Doryx

Doryx (generic name, doxycycline hyclate) is an antibiotic used for gonococcal infections. It's also available as Vibramycin and Vibra-Tabs.

Some possible side effects are pain in the chest, swelling of the face, difficulty swallowing, inflamed tongue, and genital or rectal itching. Bacteria that are not destroyed by Doryx may grow in large numbers and cause a secondary infection.

Erythromycin

Erythromycin is an antibiotic used for Lyme Disease. It is available under several brand names, including E-Mycin, ERYC, Erythrocin, Ilosone, and PCE.

Some possible side effects include nausea and vomiting, anorexia, rash, diarrhea, pain in the abdomen, as well as yellowing of the skin and eyes.

If you've had liver disease, make sure your doctor knows about it before you take this drug.

Etidronate

Etidronate is an antihypercalcemic used for Paget's Disease. Also available as Didronel and EHDP, it helps regulate bone development.

Some possible side effects include bone pain, nausea, diarrhea, and swelling of various parts of the body.

Feldene

Feldene (generic name, piroxicam) is an NSAID used for osteoarthritis and rheumatoid arthritis. It reduces joint pain, swelling, inflammation and stiffness.

Some possible side effects are abdominal pain, anemia, dizziness, nosebleed, elevated blood pressure, sweating, vomiting blood, the "blahs," headache, itching, nausea, and dizziness. See your doctor regularly to monitor for possible internal bleeding, ulcers, and so on.

Flagyl

Flagyl (generic name, metronidazole) is an antibiotic used for bone and joint infections. It's also available as Protostat.

Some possible side effects are abdominal cramps, headaches, seizures, decreased sex drive, furry tongue, inflamed rectum, pelvic pressure, and vaginal yeast infection.

Alcohol can combine with Flagyl to cause a variety of difficult side effects, so don't drink or take over-the-counter medications containing alcohol while taking this drug.

Fosamax

Fosamax (generic name, alendronate sodium) is used for Paget's disease. It helps maintain bone integrity.

Some possible side effects include pain in the joints and bones, muscle pain, difficulty swallowing, ulcers in the esophagus, diarrhea, and nausea. Be sure to ask your doctor to explain carefully when and how to take this drug.

Ibuprofen

Ibuprofen is an NSAID used for osteoarthritis, rheumatoid arthritis, juvenile rheumatoid arthritis, and Carpal Tunnel Syndrome. It's available under several names, including Advil, Motrin, and Rufen. It reduces joint pain and swelling.

Some possible side effects include headache, itching, nervousness, ringing in the ears, and abdominal problems including pain, bloating, constipation, diarrhea, and flatulence.

Motrin and Advil are available over-the-counter, without a prescription. See your doctor regularly to monitor for possible internal bleeding, ulcers, and so on.

Imuran

Imuran (generic name, azathioprine) is an immunosuppressive used for rheumatoid arthritis and systemic lupus erythematosus. It lessens the body's response to infections and interferes with the action of the white blood cells, which inadvertently causes the symptoms.

Some possible side effects include infection, suppression of the bone marrow, liver damage, baldness, skin rashes, diarrhea, nausea, and vomiting.

Indocin

Indocin (generic name, indomethacin) is an NSAID used for osteoarthritis, rheumatoid arthritis, bursitis, ankylosing spondylitis, gout, and tendonitis. It reduces joint pain, swelling, inflammation and stiffness.

Some possible side effects include hair loss, hepatitis, vaginal bleeding, depression, fatigue, dizziness, indigestion, nausea, stomach pain and upset, and vertigo. See your doctor regularly to monitor for possible internal bleeding, ulcers, and so on.

Keflex

Keflex (generic name, cephalexin hydrochloride) is an antibiotic used for infections, such as those found in infectious arthritis. It is also available as Keftab.

Some possible side effects include colitis, confusion, fatigue, fever, hallucinations, diarrhea, joint pain and inflammation, seizures, vaginal inflammation and discharge.

Lodine

Lodine (generic name, etodolac) is an NSAID used for osteoarthritis and rheumatoid arthritis. It reduces joint pain, swelling, inflammation, and stiffness.

Some possible side effects are blurred vision, chills, pain or difficulty upon urinating, more frequent urination, asthma, fever, black stools (a sign of stomach bleeding), rapid heart beat, and congestive heart failure.

See your doctor regularly to monitor for possible internal bleeding, ulcers, and so on.

Medrol

Medrol (generic name, methylprednisolone) is a corticosteroid used for rheumatoid arthritis, gout, and lupus. It reduces inflammation.

Some possible side effects include convulsions, bone fractures, bruising, irregular menstruation, fluid retention, muscle weakness and wasting, osteoporosis, and poor wound healing. This drug can increase the susceptibility to infections. It can also "hide" the presence of infections.

Miacalcin

Miacalcin (generic name, calcitonin-salmon) is a synthetic hormone used for Paget's Disease. Also available as Calcimar, it helps regulate calcium levels in bone and blood.

Some possible side effects are shock, difficulty breathing, swelling of the tongue or throat, and other signs of serious allergic reaction.

Minocin

Minocin (generic name, minocycline hydrochloride) is an antibiotic used for infections, such as those found in infectious arthritis. It's also available as Dynacin.

Some possible side effects include joint ache and inflammation, genital sores, hearing difficulties, hepatitis, hives, dizziness, skin peeling, skin eruptions, and inflammation. Minocin can cause trouble for those with existing kidney problems.

Naprosyn

Naprosyn (generic name, naproxen) is an NSAID used for osteoarthritis, rheumatoid arthritis, juvenile rheumatoid arthritis, bursitis, tendonitis, gout, and ankylosing spondylitis. It reduces joint pain, swelling, inflammation, and stiffness. It's also available as EC-Naprosyn. Some possible side effects are difficulty breathing, drowsiness, skin eruptions, blood in the urine, vomiting blood, itching, abdominal pain, bruising, and constipation. See your doctor regularly to monitor for possible internal bleeding, ulcers, and so on.

Orudis

Orudis (generic name, ketoprofen) is an NSAID used for osteoarthritis and rheumatoid arthritis. It reduces joint pain, swelling, inflammation, and stiffness. It's also available as Oruvail, Actron, and Orudis KT.

Some possible side effects are kidney damage, insomnia, nervousness, fluid retention, belching, loosening of the fingernails, impotence, flatulence, headache, and nausea. See your doctor regularly to monitor for possible internal bleeding, ulcers, and so on.

Pediapred

Pediapred (generic name, prednisolone sodium phosphate) is a steroid used for rheumatoid arthritis and gout. It reduces inflammation.

Some possible side effects are loss of bone, backbone collapse, fracture of the long bones, redness of the face, glaucoma, skin thinning, and eyeball protrusion. This drug can increase the susceptibility to infections. It can also "hide" the presence of infections.

Penicillamine

Penicillamine, also available as Cuprimine and Depen, is used for rheumatoid arthritis. We don't know exactly how penicillamine helps. It may interfere with the action of certain white blood cells that inadvertently damage joints.

Penicillamine is a slow-acting drug; two to three months may pass before its beneficial effects are felt. If and when it works, it reduces joint pain, swelling, and tenderness.

Some possible side effects include lack of appetite, swollen lymph glands, diarrhea, and skin rashes.

Penicillin

Penicillin in an antibiotic used for Lyme Disease. It's available in a variety of generic and brand names, including Bicillin, Duracillin, Pentids, Pen Vee, and Pipracil.

Some possible side effects include rashes, itching, fainting, discoloration of the tongue, nausea, diarrhea, blood in the urine, and swelling.

Plaquenil

Plaquenil (generic name, hydroxychloroquine sulfate) is an antimalarial used for rheumatoid arthritis and lupus. It reduces joint pain, swelling, inflammation, and stiffness.

Some possible side effects are changes in eye pigmentation, blind spots, difficulty focusing the eyes and other eye problems, lessened muscle coordination, hair loss, and changes in skin and hair coloration.

Don't expect instant results because Plaquenil is a slow-acting drug.

Ponstel

Ponstel (generic name, mefenamic acid) is an NSAID used for Carpal Tunnel Syndrome to reduce inflammation and moderate the pain.

Some possible side effects include abdominal pain, vomiting, nausea, diarrhea, blood in the urine, painful urination, insomnia, anorexia, kidney failure, and difficulty breathing. See your doctor regularly to monitor for possible internal bleeding, ulcers, and so on.

Relafen

Relafen (generic name, nabumetone) is an NSAID used for osteoarthritis and rheumatoid arthritis. It reduces joint pain, swelling, inflammation, and stiffness.

Some possible side effects are itching, insomnia, nervousness, constipation, diarrhea, dizziness, ringing in the ears, and stomach inflammation. See your doctor regularly to monitor for possible internal bleeding, ulcers, and so on.

Rheumatrex

Rheumatrex (generic name methotrexate) is an anticancer drug used for rheumatoid arthritis when other drugs have not helped. It may slow the errant immune system reaction that is causing problems.

Some possible side effects include mouth ulcers, the "blahs," dizziness, fatigue, abdominal pain and distress, fever, chills, impotence, diabetes, and greater susceptibility to infections.

Ridaura

Ridaura (generic name, auranofin) is a gold preparation used for rheumatoid arthritis. It reduces or eliminates swelling of the joints.

Some possible side effects can include abnormalities of the blood cells, anemia, bronchitis, sores in the mouth, pinkeye, metallic taste, diarrhea, loss of appetite, flatulence, and vomiting.

Most gold compounds are injected, but Ridaura is taken orally. It is usually given only after NSAIDs have not helped. It's a slow-acting medication, so don't expect quick results.

Sandimmune

Sandimmune (generic name, cyclosporine) is an immunosuppressant used for severe cases of rheumatoid arthritis.

Some possible side effects are elevated blood pressure, kidney damage, growth of the gums, tremor, convulsions, coughing, acne, tumor of the lymph system, difficulty breathing, and joint or muscle pain. Sandimmune suppresses the immune system, making you susceptible to other diseases, including cancer.

The amount of cyclosporine absorbed from Sandimmune varies from person to person, so your doctor will need to check the levels in your blood regularly.

Sulfinpyrazone

Sulfinpyrazone is an antigout medication available under brand names such as Antazone, Anturan, Anturane and Novopyrazone. It works by lowering uric acid levels.

Some possible side effects are difficulty urinating, nausea, low back pain, and rash.

Tegison

Tegison (generic name, etretinate) is used for psoriatic arthritis. It reduces inflammation and improves psoriatic lesions and scaliness of the skin.

Some possible side effects include pain in the bones and joints, dry eyes and skin, nosebleeds, muscle cramps, loss of hearing, and fetal abnormalities if taken while pregnant.

Tegison is given to patients who don't respond well to other forms of treatment. It may take up to a month to begin working.

Tetracycline

Tetracycline is an antibiotic used for Lyme Disease. There are many generic and brand name tetracyclines, including Doryx, doxycycline, methacycline, minocycline, Sumycin, and Vibramycin.

Some possible side effects are hives, itching, sore mouth, nausea, vomiting, vaginal discharge, dark tongue, rectal and genital itching, faintness, anemia, brownish-yellowing of the skin and teeth, and skin sensitivity to sunlight.

Tolectin

Tolectin (generic name tolmetin sodium) is an NSAID used for osteoarthritis, rheumatoid arthritis, and juvenile rheumatoid arthritis. It reduces joint pain, swelling, inflammation, and stiffness.

Some possible side effects are weight changes, weakness, elevated blood pressure, hives, kidney failure, urinary tract infections, painful urination, and dizziness.

This drug is used for both short-term and long-term treatment of the previously-mentioned diseases. Tolectin can damage the liver, kidney, and eyes, and increase bleeding time. See your doctor regularly to monitor for these problems as well as possible internal bleeding, ulcers, and so on.

Trilisate

Trilisate (generic name, choline magnesium trisalicylate) is an NSAID used for osteoarthritis, rheumatoid arthritis, and juvenile rheumatoid arthritis.

Some possible side effects are stomach pain, heartburn, vomiting, constipation, and diarrhea.

Trilisate may be linked to Reye's Syndrome, a serious ailment. See your doctor regularly to monitor for this problem, as well as for possible internal bleeding, ulcers, and so on.

Tylenol

Tylenol (generic name, acetaminophen) is used for joint and muscle pain. It is also available as Aspirin-Free Anacin and Panadol.

Some possible side effects include indications of an allergic reaction such as hives, swelling, and difficulty breathing.

Vioxx

See Chapter 23.

Voltaren

Voltaren (generic name diclofenac sodium) is an NSAID used for osteoarthritis, rheumatoid arthritis, and ankylosing spondylitis. It reduces joint pain, swelling, inflammation, and stiffness. It's also available as Voltaren-XR and Cataflam (diclofenac potassium).

Some possible side effects are diarrhea, itching, cramps, constipation, ringing in the ears, and rash.

Voltaren-XR is used for long-term treatment. Tell your doctor if you have kidney or heart problems, or elevated blood pressure. Then see your doctor regularly to monitor for these and other problems, including internal bleeding, ulcers, and so on.

Zyloprim

Zyloprim (generic name, allopurinol) is used to reduce uric acid production in gout. It's also available as Lopurin.

Some possible side effects are chills, fever, diarrhea, attacks of gout, rash, itch, stomach pain and other problems, and headache.

Zyloprim does not stop gout attacks that have already begun — it's a long-term treatment for reducing symptoms of recurring attacks.

Chapter 8

Cuts That Cure: Surgeries for Arthritis

● ●

In This Chapter

▶ Deciding whether you may be a candidate for joint surgery

▶ Understanding the role of the orthopedic surgeon

▶ Learning about the different types of joint surgery

▶ Finding out how to prepare for surgery

▶ Making preparations for a post-surgical recovery

● ●

*T*he idea of having surgery is always a scary one. Any time you allow a surgeon to ply his trade on your body, you are taking certain risks, some great and others small. But under the right conditions, surgery performed on a diseased joint can bring results that are nothing short of spectacular. Pain can be reduced or eliminated, range of motion restored, deformities corrected, and joint function vastly improved. Still, surgery is not for everybody. Whether it's right for you depends on many factors.

When Do You Need Surgery?

While your doctor can tell you all about what goes on inside your body, only *you* know what's going on inside your head. Do a little soul-searching to determine whether you really want and need the surgery by asking yourself the following questions:

✔ Is the pain interfering with my ability to lead a productive and satisfying life?

✔ Do I rely on pain relievers taken at the maximum allowable dosage to get through the day?

> ✔ Have I tried all other pain-relieving methods (physical therapy, exercise, pain management strategies, and so on) without success?
>
> ✔ Are my expectations of the surgery results realistic?
>
> ✔ Will I participate fully in my postsurgery rehabilitation?

If you can answer "yes" to all of these questions, you may be mentally and emotionally ready to undergo joint surgery.

The Orthopedic Surgeon

If you're considering surgical treatment for your arthritis, you need to consult with an *orthopedic surgeon (orthopedist),* the kind of doctor who specializes in treating diseases of the muscles, bones, and joints. An orthopedic surgeon is trained in both surgical and nonsurgical methods. *Nonsurgical treatments* consist of casting, splinting, and joint injections. *Surgical treatments* include removal of the joint lining, cutting and resetting of the bone, bone fusion, and joint reconstruction. *Arthroscopic surgery,* a special technique that has gained great popularity in recent years, is the one of many techniques in the orthopedic surgeon's repertoire.

Your family physician or internist may be able to refer you to a competent orthopedic surgeon, but don't automatically assume that this person is the right choice for you. Review the suggestions in Chapter 5 for finding a doctor and apply them in your current search.

Questions to Ask Your Doctor before Undergoing Surgery

Because surgery is a drastic and (at least somewhat) risky option, you shouldn't consider it until all other measures have been exhausted. First, you and your doctor should thoroughly investigate and make use of the many nonsurgical options, such as medications, diet, physical therapy, pain management strategies, exercise, and alternative methods. The truth of the matter is that most people do not need surgery to manage their arthritis.

In some cases, though, surgery can be a godsend. When rheumatic finger joints render your hands nearly useless, or when a painful, osteoarthritic hip makes walking out to the mailbox a major feat, certain surgical procedures may be able to give you a new lease on life.

Is surgery an option?

Whether a surgery succeeds depends on two things: the condition itself and the body in question. Some disease states respond wonderfully to surgery, while others show little or no improvement. People are like that, too. One person may come through a surgical procedure with flying colors, zip through recovery, and be thrilled with the results. Another person, equally affected and undergoing an identical surgery, may become trapped in a long, drawn-out recovery period that garners less-than-optimal results. Putting it simply, surgery is a highly individual matter and may or may not be best for you. To find out, begin by asking your orthopedic surgeon the following questions:

- **Do my symptoms and my test results go hand-in-hand?** In other words, can your doctor confirm your diagnosis? You certainly don't want to undergo surgery for a problem that may not exist.

- **Does my kind of arthritis respond well to surgery?** Surgery is most often performed on those with rheumatoid arthritis or incapacitating osteoarthritis, while it's rarely the treatment-of-choice for gout, sclero-derma or lupus. Those with ankylosing spondylitis are "iffy" candidates for surgery: Sometimes surgery is used to straighten their spines or replace joints, but excessive bone growth can complicate the recovery process.

- **Is the surgery a permanent fix for my symptoms or will it have to be redone eventually?** A shoulder joint replacement is considered a one-time event; but a knee or hip replacement may have to be redone in 10 to 20 years. This fact is important in the timing of the surgery. Hip replacements, for example, are often done on people age 60 or older because they generally don't outlive the implant. But a 50 year-old with a bad hip may be encouraged to "hang on" for another 5 or 10 years before getting a replacement, because revision surgeries often involve added complications.

- **What results can I expect from this surgery?** In other words, what is the surgery going to do for you? How will it affect your pain, your range of motion, and the stability of your joint(s)? What kind of activities will you be able to participate in after you recover? What limitations will you have?

- **What risks are involved?** Make sure the doctor explains all the compli-cations that can result from the surgery (for example, infection, nerve damage, and so on), as well as the risks involved in undergoing the surgery itself (such as cardiac arrest).

- **What is involved in the postsurgery rehabilitation?** Rehabilitation can be a long, sometimes painful process that usually requires your utmost dedication and hard work. Be sure you know what lies ahead before you consent to surgery. If you're not willing to do the work, the outcome of your surgery may be compromised.

✓ **Am I physically able to withstand the surgery?** It is common practice to have a physical examination before surgery to make sure you and your body are up to it. The condition of your heart, respiratory system, blood, and overall health will be taken into account when assessing whether you can withstand the rigors of surgery.

✓ **What does the future hold if I don't have surgery?** If you are already in great pain, finding out that it will get worse unless you have the surgery may tip the scales for you in favor of the procedure. Fortunately, you can often put off arthritis surgery indefinitely without compromising its effectiveness.

Types of Joint Surgery

Because the joint is an intricate piece of "machinery," and many different things can go wrong with it, joint surgery is complex and wide-ranging. It can involve flushing the joint with water, resurfacing rough bone ends or cartilage, cutting away inflamed membranes, growing bone where it otherwise wouldn't be, and even taking the whole joint out and starting from scratch with a new one.

Removal of diseased joint lining (synovectomy)

People who have rheumatoid arthritis may benefit from having a synovectomy, in which the surgeon removes an inflamed, overgrown joint lining (synovium).

In rheumatoid arthritis, the inflamed, thickened synovium can overgrow to the point that it invades the joint's supporting structures — the bones, cartilage, muscles, and ligaments. This growth can cause damage to the joint over time. At the same time, the synovium releases enzymes that cause bone and cartilage to breakdown. Removing the offending lining stops the synovial invasion and reduces the amount of destructive enzymes released.

The surgeon may make a large incision that exposes the entire joint. Or, in the case of arthroscopic surgery, tiny incisions may be made that are just large enough to accommodate the insertion of an arthroscope (a flexible tube about as big around as a pencil that's used for diagnostic and surgical purposes). In either procedure, the joint lining is cut away, leaving just enough behind to produce lubricating fluid. Recovery can take several weeks.

Pain relief and protection against joint destruction can last for a couple of years, so more radical treatments, such as joint replacement, can be postponed.

This type of surgery is not a permanent cure, as the synovium eventually grows back.

Cutting and resetting the bone (osteotomy)

To perform an osteotomy, the surgeon removes a section of bone to correct joint alignment. (*Osteo* is the Greek word for *bone; tomy* means *to cut.*) Those suffering from osteoarthritis, especially of the knee, and ankylosing spondylitis can benefit from this surgery. It's also helpful for joints that are wearing improperly but still have a healthy area.

A misaligned joint can cause uneven wearing on the bones and cartilage as well as general joint pain. After proper alignment is restored, the force exerted on the joint is distributed more evenly. Excess pressure is released from cartilage and bone, "worn spots" have the chance to repair themselves, and pain is reduced.

If the patient is suffering from osteoarthritis, a slice or wedge of bone is surgically removed, allowing the joint to realign. The "raw edges" of the bone are connected with screws and eventually grow together again. If the patient has ankylosing spondylitis, the spinal disease, the damaged tissue and bone that lock the spine into its unnatural, "bent-over" position are removed so that the spine can return to its natural, upright position.

Pain relief, improved joint function, increased range of motion, and greater joint stability are the benefits of this type of surgery.

Recovery may take anywhere from six to twelve months, but there is a possibility that joint function may not improve. Alterations in joint alignment can make future joint replacements difficult. For many, the benefits last only a few years.

Fusing the bone (arthrodesis)

Folks who suffer from rheumatoid arthritis may benefit from having certain bones fused. The surgeon positions the joint into its most functional alignment and then "locks" it in place permanently.

This surgery helps to stabilize and relieve pain in highly unsteady and painful joints. Arthrodesis is primarily performed on the spine but also can be used on the thumb, hip, knee, and wrist when replacement is either not feasible or has already proved unsuccessful. Fusion of the hip joint may be required for those who need a total hip replacement but can't have one, either because their bones aren't healthy enough or because they are too young and/or too active. (Hip replacements typically last only about ten- fifteen years, and second replacements often don't work as well.) Fusion of the thumb joint can make grasping possible. Fusion of the knee is sometimes done when a knee replacement becomes infected and won't "take," while the wrist may be fused because it's a highly unstable joint and very difficult to replace.

The surgeon removes cartilage from the opposing bone ends and also removes a surface layer of bone. The joint is positioned in the way in which it can be of greatest use, and then the bone ends are joined using pins, rods or screws. Splinting or casting helps keep the joint stable, while new bone growth fuses it permanently into place.

The surgery helps to relieve pain and can increase the ability to use the joint (in a limited way). Although joint motion is forfeited with arthrodesis, joint function improves. A person with a fused hip, for example, *can* walk, even if it is with a limp, which may be progress for one who is otherwise wheelchair-bound. Recovery from this surgery can take several months.

Rebuilding the joint (arthroplasty)

Those who suffer from severe, chronic osteoarthritis and rheumatoid arthritis may benefit from this type of surgery. The surgeon reconstructs the joint using artificial parts, as well as some of the existing natural tissues. The hip and knee are the most commonly replaced joints, but ankles, shoulders, elbows, and knuckles are also done routinely and successfully.

Sometimes a joint degenerates to the point where the pain is severe or constant and function is seriously impaired. By surgically removing the old, diseased joint and replacing it with a new, man-made one, pain is relieved and mobility is restored.

With the patient under anesthesia, the surgeon opens the joint and detaches the tendons and ligaments from the bone. He dislocates the joint, and cuts away the diseased or weakened parts of the bone. The surgeon uses plastic and/or metal prostheses to replace the missing parts of the joint and may cement them into place. He then fits the joint parts together, reattaches ligaments and tendons, and closes the incision. (See the sidebar on hip replacement.)

How doctors perform a total hip replacement

A ball-and-socket joint that sometimes bears as much as ten times the weight of the body, the hip must provide a secure anchor between the pelvis and thigh bone (*femur*) if it's to do its job. In a partial hip replacement, either the ball or the socket is replaced with an artificial structure. In a total hip replacement, both are replaced. The total hip replacement is done in several stages:

The tendons and ligaments that are connected to the femur's ball-shaped end are carefully detached.

The hip joint is dislocated, in order to separate the pelvis and femur.

The ball-shaped end is cut away from the femur.

A special tool is used to hollow out the socket, so that it will be large enough to hold the new socket, a cup-like structure made of a kind of plastic called polyethylene.

The plastic socket is cemented into place using joint compound.

A shaft is cut down the center of the femur. A metal ball with a rod attached (it looks like a door knob with a root) is inserted in the shaft and cemented into place.

The metal ball is inserted into the plastic socket, the ligaments and tendons repaired, and the wound is closed.

In the majority of cases, joint replacements provide pain relief, restored mobility, and improved joint stability. In the case of the weight-bearing joints, such as the hip or knee, this improved function can restore not only a patient's independence but also his or her overall outlook on life. There are complications, however. Infection at the site of the surgery may require removal of the implant; the prosthesis can loosen; or the joint may dislocate. Replacements of weight-bearing joints can wear out — hips only last ten-fifteen years, while knees may last as long as twenty — and when joint replacements wear out, the surgery must be repeated. (A shoulder replacement, however, can last for life.) Other complications of joint replacement include blood clots (especially in the leg), damage to the nerves surrounding the replacement, and legs that are unequal in length.

If you're planning on having a knee replacement, you may think it's a good idea to replace both knees at once and save yourself some time and money. But studies show that those undergoing double knee replacements are more likely to suffer from serious complications (dislocation, inflammation, nerve damage, and so on) than those who take it one step (or one knee) at a time.

You have a much better chance of enjoying a successful hip or knee replacement if you exercise, stay away from high-impact sports and activities, maintain your ideal body weight, and guard against infection.

Figure 8-1:
In a total hip replacement, the hip socket is replaced with a cup-like structure made of polyethylene, and the head of the femur is replaced with a metal ball attached to a rod.

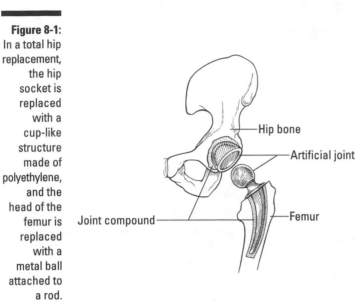

Hip bone

Artificial joint

Joint compound

Femur

With cement or without?

Over time, the cement used in hip replacements can begin to crack and break into little pieces, causing the prosthesis to loosen. These wayward little pieces of cement can take fragments of bone with them as they fall away, weakening and degrading the overall bone structure. Because of this, some people opt for *cementless* hip replacements. The ball-and-stem part of the cementless prosthesis has a rough, bumpy outer skin, like a horned toad, that causes bone to grow into the spaces between the bumps, securing the real bone to the artificial part.

Advantages of cementless replacements:

✔ This type of replacement may last longer because there is no cement to crack and break away.

✔ Revision surgery can be easier to do.

Disadvantages of cementless replacements:

✔ Recovery can take a long time, with activity limited for as much as three months while bone "grows into" the replacement part.

✔ Soft or porous bones may not be able to bond tightly enough to the prosethesis to allow a successful cementless hip replacement.

✔ It's hard to get a perfect fit — 10 to 20 percent of patients experience pain in the thigh that is sometimes severe.

Transplanting cartilage (autologous chondrocyte implantation)

Osteoarthritis sufferers (especially in those under 40 who have experienced trauma to the joint) benefit from this procedure.

For this procedure, the surgeon takes healthy cartilage cells from one part of the body and transplants them into a joint with damaged cartilage. These transplanted cells continue to grow, producing a new, healthier cartilage that eventually replaces the old.

When a joint suffers trauma, the *chondrocytes* (cartilage-producing cells) change the way they act. They may make smaller amounts of certain cartilage components *(proteoglycans* and *collagen),* while churning out more of the enzymes that break down the cartilage. This decrease in the building up of cartilage, plus an increase in cartilage destruction, adds up to damaged, poor-quality tissue. But if the old chondrocytes can be replaced with new chondrocytes that work properly, production and maintenance of healthy cartilage may be restored.

The surgeon harvests healthy cartilage cells from another area in the body (not the damaged joint) and mixes them together with a special solution that includes some fluid taken from the patient. The cells are carefully cultured in a laboratory for a few weeks, where they grow and multiply. Then these cells are injected into the patient's damaged joint, where they take hold and begin to grow new cartilage. Because the cells and fluid come from the patient's own body, there is less chance of rejection.

The surgery helps with pain relief and restored mobility through a relatively non-invasive method.

The cost of the surgery is very high (as much as $40,000), and few insurance companies will pay for the procedure. Because this is a new approach, no one knows how long the new cartilage will last.

Getting Ready for Surgery

Careful preparation for surgery helps ensure the best possible results. Your tasks include the following:

- ✔ Getting yourself into the best possible physical shape
- ✔ Arranging adequate postoperative care
- ✔ Finding someone who can take over your responsibilities for as long as necessary

- ✔ Resolving insurance and money matters
- ✔ Setting up a recovery plan with your doctor

Get yourself into the best possible physical shape

Prepare for your surgery as if you were an athlete training for a competition. Eat highly nutritious meals, exercise regularly (if you're up to it), get plenty of sleep, and stay away from alcohol or unnecessary drugs. Surgery is done carefully, utilizing every precaution, but it is still a major assault on the body. The better your health going in, the better your body can withstand the trauma and the faster you'll recover.

Your doctor will undoubtedly give you several presurgical instructions. You may be asked to wash with a special soap or take a course of antibiotics. Most certainly you'll be asked to avoid taking certain drugs that can thin the blood and increase bleeding time.

Arrange adequate postoperative care

You'll need someone to take you home from the hospital, someone who can take care of you for the next several days, and someone who can help around the house for at least a week or two, depending on the extent of your surgery. You may have an angel in your life who can play all three roles, or you may have to call on a variety of friends and family members. One thing is sure: You can't do it alone.

Find someone who can handle your responsibilities

If you are undergoing major surgery on a weight-bearing joint, you may be at least partially out of commission for months. Driving, shopping, taking care of children, doing housework, and or going to work may be impossible for you for quite some time. It's essential that you have a solid support system in place. The last thing you need is to be forced into doing things that are beyond your capabilities.

Resolve financial and insurance matters

Before your surgery, it's imperative that you find out exactly what your insurance company will cover and how much of the tab you'll be expected to pick up. The stress of unexpected medical expenses is extremely disruptive mentally and emotionally, and can be a major hindrance to your recovery.

Make a recovery plan with your doctor

Although no one can predict exactly when you'll pass certain milestones on the road to recovery, it will ease your mind and give you something to look forward to if you have a list of the progressive steps of healing. Ask your doctor to help you construct a recovery plan that maps out these steps. Studies show that people recover faster and more completely if they have a good idea of what to expect both during and after surgery.

Chapter 9

Overcoming the Ouch: Strategies for Pain Management

In This Chapter

▶ Understanding the causes of arthritis pain

▶ Breaking the pain cycle

▶ Exploring noninvasive ways to control pain

*I*t's hard to be happy when you hurt. Pain has a way of enveloping your mind, hijacking your brain, and making it difficult to concentrate on work, family, hobbies, or anything else. You desperately want to be fully involved in life, but the pain distracts, worries, irritates, and depresses you to the point where you can think of little else. The things that you used to do with ease can suddenly become difficult or even impossible to accomplish. Living with long-standing chronic pain can wear you down, exhaust you, depress you, and make you feel that life isn't worth living. Fortunately, there are plenty of strategies (both physical and mental) that can help you cope with pain. So even if your pain isn't completely banished, you *can* release its stranglehold on your life.

In this chapter, we focus on physical strategies for managing the pain. (See Chapter 13 for mental pain-management strategies.)

What Causes Arthritis Pain?

Arthritis pain comes in many forms: stabbing, aching, twisting, burning, pressing, stretching, and crushing. Some people describe it as "killing," "a fire," "a knife that someone keeps jabbing into me," "a bowling ball knocking the pins down over and over," "a continual car wreck," and "something I wouldn't even wish on my worst enemy."

Several things can cause the pain of arthritis. For example, it may result from something about the disease process itself, such as

- **Inflammation:** Swollen, hot, inflamed joint tissues.
- **Joint damage:** Bones grinding against each other, tendons that have slipped, joint misalignment or loosening, invasion of the bone by the synovium (joint lining), and so on.

Your arthritis pain may also be related to your body's response to the disease. For example:

- **Muscle tension:** Tensing up as a reaction to your pain can spread pain to the muscles and make everything feel worse.
- **Strained muscles and supporting tissues:** When overcompensating for an injured area, you can unintentionally put excessive stress on a different area.
- **Fatigue:** Feeling dragged out due to illness can make your pain even more intense and difficult to cope with.

Of course, when you're hurting, it doesn't matter much whether your pain is caused by or related to the arthritis. You just want it to stop! But for many people, the pain just seems to go on and on — and on.

Acute Pain Versus Chronic Pain

The kind of pain you feel when you touch a hot stove, called acute pain, is absolutely vital to your well-being. *Acute pain* is a warning that you've injured yourself and need to do something about it — now! Acute pain is episodic, meaning that it comes on quickly, builds rapidly to a crescendo, then tapers off and disappears. Suppose, for example, that you fall down and skin your knee. It really hurts! But, by the time you wash, disinfect, and bandage the area, your pain is already receding and will soon disappear entirely. Your reaction to acute pain has served its purpose. Although acute pain can be excruciating, at least it has a purpose and an end.

Chronic pain, however, is another story. Like a barrage of telegrams repeating the same message over and over, chronic pain is no longer a useful warning; instead, it's an agonizing, debilitating tirade. Resistant to medical treatment, chronic pain can become the constantly tormenting drumbeat underlying your every activity, day and night. Bam! Bam! Bam! It won't let up. Not surprisingly, the number one cause of chronic pain is arthritis.

The pain cycle

Many arthritis sufferers become extremely frustrated and depressed by pain and the decline in their physical abilities. Unfortunately, stress and depression can and do make pain worse, setting the *pain cycle* into motion. The physical pain from arthritis causes stress and upset about the lost physical abilities. This, in turn, can trigger muscle tension that worsens the pain and further limits physical activities, causing even more stress and depression; thus, the cycle continues.

Happily, there are many great things you can do to break the pain cycle and live more comfortably, even if your pain is chronic. The key is to block the pain signals moving through your nerves and spinal cord, which prevents them from registering in the brain. The medicines discussed in Chapter 7 can eliminate a little or a lot of your hurting. With medication plus the pain management methods that we describe in this chapter and the next, you should be able to block many of these signals and manage your arthritis pain. The key word here is manage. *Managing* chronic pain means reducing its severity and decreasing it to the point where you can get on with your life, not eradicating it completely.

Dealing with chronic pain syndrome

You usually don't have to worry much about dealing with acute pain. It certainly hurts, but often responds well to medicine and doesn't wear out its welcome. Getting rid of acute pain is typically your doctor's job. Dealing with chronic pain, however, is a different matter.

The goal in chronic pain management is to block pain messages before they reach the brain. There are several natural ways you can try, apart from using drugs. For example:

- Exercise that's appropriate to your condition
- Hot or cold treatments
- Water therapy
- Massage
- Magnets
- Topical pain releivers
- Relaxation
- TENS (transcutaneous electrical stimulation)

On the other hand, several "natural" things can make your pain even worse:

- ✔ Anxiety
- ✔ Depression
- ✔ Fatigue
- ✔ Focusing on your pain
- ✔ Physical overexertion
- ✔ Progression of the disease
- ✔ Stress

Your treatment team

Chronic pain is a complex phenomenon that involves the original or on-going disease process, the way your body deals with the problem mechanically, and your mental and emotional responses. A team of professionals, each with their own expertise, best handles this multifaceted problem. People whom you may want to be a part of your treatment team include

- ✔ **Your doctor:** To guide your treatment and prescribe medication, if necessary.
- ✔ **A physical therapist:** To help you build strength and restore range of motion. (See "What does a physical therapist do?" on page 10.)
- ✔ **An occupational therapist:** To teach you how to overcome limitations, place less strain on your joints when performing daily activities, and prevent further damage.
- ✔ **An exercise physiologist:** To help you devise an exercise program that will increase strength, flexibility, and endurance without putting undue strain on your joints. (This is also a function of the physical therapist, whose services may be paid for by insurance.)
- ✔ **A psychologist:** To help you cope with depression, anger, and/or other emotional issues.
- ✔ **A pharmacist:** To offer advice on the proper use of medication.
- ✔ **A social worker:** To recommend support groups or other special services.

You can also visit pain management clinics that have such teams already assembled for you. Although some of these clinics specialize in treating specific types of pain, there are others that treat all types. (Insurance coverage varies according to plan, and you'll probably need a referral from your doctor.) For a pain clinic in your area, contact one of the organizations listed under Pain Management in Appendix B of this book.

MEDICAL SPEAK

Controlling pain the natural way

Your body makes certain substances that can decrease or even block pain sensations, as well as others that can increase your pain. The pain blockers include *endorphins* and *enkephalins*, substances that can slow or stop nerve cells from firing and sending pain messages to the brain. These chemicals are so powerful, their effects are often compared to those of morphine. Naturally, you want to produce more endorphins and enkephalins when you're in pain. You also want to have plenty of the brain hormone serotonin and other substances that play a role in manufacturing and releasing these internal painkillers.

Natural irritants — substances that increase the neurons' sensitivity to pain — are the flip side of the body's natural pain blockers. These irritants include *lactic acid, potassium ions, Substance P* plus the stress hormones *noradrenaline* and *norepinephrine*. Most of the pain control process revolves around increasing the production of the pain blockers while decreasing the production of the pain-intensifiers. For example, massage can increase the production of endorphins while helping the body dispense with excessive amounts of lactic acid.

Managing Your Pain

The three approaches to managing pain are

- ✔ Noninvasive methods
- ✔ Medication
- ✔ Surgery

Noninvasive methods

These methods are physical and/or psychological treatments that don't intrude on or cause harm to the body. They are the least-traumatic approaches to pain management.

Hot and cold packs, massage, ultrasound, joint manipulation, magnets, splints, and supports are all noninvasive pain relief techniques, because they don't involve cutting, puncturing, or otherwise traumatizing the body. Other noninvasive techniques include psychotherapy, self-hypnosis, deep breathing, progressive relaxation, creative imagery, and biofeedback. (See Chapter 13 for more on these mental strategies for pain relief.)

At best, noninvasive approaches to pain management are very helpful; at worst they're probably harmless. With no side effects, incisions, blood loss, addiction potential, or other hazards, these techniques should certainly be thoroughly explored by you and your doctor before you move on to the harsher, more dangerous methods of pain relief.

Medications

From mild aspirin to powerful DMARDS (See Chapter 7), medicines can be beneficial but risky. In certain situations, the doctor may recommend injecting substances like corticosteroids right into the afflicted area.

As we point out in Chapter 7, NSAIDS and analgesics are the most commonly prescribed painkillers for arthritis, and your doctor may also prescribe antidepressants if emotional lows are a problem. But, like most medications, painkillers and/or antidepressants have their pros and cons. Although they can be helpful initially, long-term use can cause stomach problems and/or drug dependence. And, over time, their effectiveness can start to wane.

Surgery

Surgery, which involves the making of an incision and the manipulation of the inner workings of the body, is always a risky, traumatic procedure.

Undergoing surgery to relieve pain can produce dramatic results in some cases, but it always carries serious risks and side-effects, ranging from infection to death. Consider surgery only as a last resort. (See Chapter 8 for a complete discussion of the surgeries for arthritis.)

Most pain treatment programs begin with the least traumatic methods, moving on to medications and/or surgery only when gentler treatments aren't successful.

Noninvasive Pain Relieving Therapies

Remember getting sick when you were a child? Your mother probably had a whole bag of tricks that could make you feel better: a cool cloth on your forehead, a warm bath, letting you lie in her bed to watch television, chamomile tea, and so on. Her methods were just simple little things, but they really *did* make you feel better.

You may be surprised at how much relief you can get from your arthritis pain by adopting the following equally simple physical strategies. Although these techniques will not *cure* your arthritis (the relief is temporary), often any respite from the pain is welcome, no matter how brief! So, next time your arthritis pain flares, try some of the following methods.

Applying heat

Warmth encourages expansion of the blood vessels, bringing more blood to the painful area and stimulating the healing process. It also helps your muscles relax, which may be just what you need if the pain you experience makes you tighten up. You can use hot packs, heating pads, heat lamps with infrared bulbs, electric blankets, or hot paraffin wax treatments to rev up your circulation, encourage overall relaxation, and make you feel better.

Another way to apply heat is to wrap yourself in a flannel sheet or a throw blanket that you've just popped into the clothes dryer for a few minutes. Although the heat won't last long, it's very cozy!

Ultrasound is a more high-tech way of accomplishing the same thing as old-fashioned heat packs. High-frequency sound waves are aimed at the affected area producing deep tissue heat, which increases circulation and promotes muscle relaxation.

Be careful not to damage your skin when applying heat. Follow these rules to protect yourself:

- ✔ Limit heat applications to no longer than 30 minutes in one area.

- ✔ Wrap the hot pack or heating pad in towels to insulate it; don't place the source of heat directly on your skin.

- ✔ To avoid steam burns or skin reactions, make sure that your skin is dry and that you haven't applied lotion or cream to it (particularly deep-heating creams).

- ✔ Inspect the area every five minutes for purplish-red skin, hives, or blisters, which are signs of skin damage.

- ✔ Allow your skin temperature to return to normal before reapplying heat.

Heat may make some conditions worse. Check with your doctor in advance to see if heat treatments are appropriate for you.

Hot paraffin wax treatments

Hot paraffin wax treatments are a nice, comfortable way to warm up painful joints in your hands and/or feet. These treatments sustain their warmth because they use wax as insulation. A physical therapist usually applies hot paraffin wax treatments, but you can also do it yourself at home.

How do hot paraffin wax treatments work? Your painful hand or foot is repeatedly dipped into a blend of melted wax and mineral oil and allowed to cool in between immersions so that the wax can harden. When the build-up is thick enough, your hand/foot is wrapped in plastic and covered with towels to preserve the heat. The locked-in warmth can be very soothing to your stiff, painful fingers or toes. After 20 minutes or so, the wrapping comes off, and the wax is peeled away.

As an added bonus, you'll find that hot paraffin wax treatments leave your skin wonderfully soft!

Don't use this treatment if your hand or foot shows any signs of skin damage.

Applying cold

Cold packs are used to reduce inflammation, ease muscle spasms, and block pain signals by numbing the affected area. Although blood flow to the chilled area is temporarily reduced, cold applications will eventually *increase* circulation, acting much like hot packs. Ice is the usual medium used to numb painful areas, but you may find it more convenient to use cold packs containing chemical mixtures that thaw slowly and don't drip.

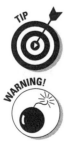

A bag of frozen peas makes a good cold pack because you can mold it around any shape, unlike a block of ice or bulky cubes. But make sure that you put the bag inside an airtight plastic bag and wrap it in a towel, because it will drip.

Watch for icy dangers and protect your skin and other tissues when using cold packs, by following these steps:

- ✔ Limit treatment to no more than twenty minutes.

- ✔ Remove the cold pack once the area is numb.

- ✔ Be on the lookout for skin damage — redness, white patches, and so on.

- ✔ Avoid cold packs if you have Raynaud's, poor circulation, sensitivity to cold, nerve damage, a lack of sensation, or heart problems.

In general, if inflammation is present, use cold; if not, use hot, although many doctors recommend that you use whatever feels good to you. The best advice is to consult your doctor before using either method.

Water therapy

Ah, what feels better than easing your stiff, sore body into a nice warm bath? The ancient Romans evidently agreed, building several health resorts throughout their wide-ranging empire for the express purpose bathing. Most notable was in the town of Bath, England, where people with arthritis came from far and wide to "take the waters."

Warm showers, baths, and whirlpools can help ease your stiffness and make you feel better. Warm water therapy is also a good way to warm up your muscles before an exercise session, relaxing them and making movement easier.

Cool water can also help, especially when inflammation is present. Immersing a painful, swollen joint in cool water or using cool compresses is a milder, less jolting version of applying an ice pack.

Pool exercises are also an extremely effective form of water therapy. Because water supports your body, exercising in a pool is like exercising in a weightless environment. With the tiresome pull of gravity greatly reduced in water, your joints can rest even as your muscles are put through a real workout. Because water provides resistance, your muscles have to work harder to perform a movement in water than they do on land. This combination adds up to more effective exercise, with less wear and tear on your joints. (See Chapter 11 for more on water exercise.)

Whether warm or cool, water can be used in a variety of ways to help ease your pain, including

- Cool hand and/or foot baths
- Cool moist compresses
- Drinking warm tea
- Warm full-body baths
- Warm hand and/or foot baths
- Warm, moist compresses
- Warm showers
- Whirlpool baths

What does a physical therapist do?

Described as a combination of buddy, drill sergeant, cheerleader, and workout partner, the physical therapist works with you to help increase your range of motion, reduce your pain, build strength, and decrease disability. "The hardest part is getting the patient to do exercises that remind them that they can't move like they used to," said Kari, a physical therapist in San Diego, California. "That seems to make them angrier and more depressed than feeling the pain does. But my job is to keep pushing, because that's the only way anybody gets better."

The physical therapist takes you through a series of exercises designed to get your joints lubed and stretch your range of movement. Joint manipulation and massage are also important parts of the physical therapy session. Perhaps most importantly, the physical therapist helps you stamp out procrastination and get to work!

Topical pain relievers

There are many topical creams, lotions, rubs, and sprays that can help with chronic arthritis pain. They typically contain one or more of the following ingredients:

✔ *Capsaicin:* A substance derived from chili peppers that decreases the nerves' concentration of "substance P" in the painful area, thus reducing pain.

✔ *Irritants:* Menthol, camphor, and other substances that produce feelings of heat, cold, or itching. These distract you from the sensation of pain.

✔ *Salicylates:* Aspirin-like compounds that desensitize nerve endings.

Topical pain relievers are usually safe and at least somewhat effective. If you decide to use them, make sure you don't apply them to broken skin, and watch for signs of skin irritation.

Joint manipulation

Joint manipulation is also known as *passive movement* because something other than your own energy is moving your joints for you. That "something" is usually a physical therapist. During joint manipulation, the physical therapist uses his or her hands to move your joints through their range of motion. Then, by applying pressure (stretching) or simply moving the joint back and forth or around and around (depending upon the joint type), the therapist can help loosen up your joints. Joint manipulation must be done carefully, however, and never overdone. Otherwise, your joints can become even more irritated and painful.

Remember, in most cases some joint movement is absolutely necessary. People with arthritis have a tendency to guard their stiff, sore joints by moving them as little as possible. Unfortunately, this can be the worst thing for them. When the joints are held still, they aren't being lubricated or nourished, their supporting muscles become weaker, circulation decreases, and ligaments and tendons tighten up, losing their resilience. Over time, an immobile joint can actually become frozen into position. That's why it's so important to keep moving your joints, whether they hurt or not. Even splinted joints should be moved, at least a little, every day.

Splints and supports

Splints are designed to support and immobilize an injured or inflamed joint. A molded piece of metal or plastic is strapped to the affected area and then wrapped with elastic bandages. You can find splints for the wrist, fingers, hands, ankles, knees, back, and neck. Splints are widely available in off-the-rack varieties or can be custom made by taking an impression of your joint and then molding heat-sensitive material to replicate the shape. Splints help to

✔ Provide support, stability, protection, and rest for injured or inflamed joints.

✔ Immobilize a joint after surgical fusion (arthrodesis) and allow healing.

✔ Ease pain during arthritis flares, although they're only temporary measures.

✔ Keep inflammation under control.

✔ Correct or prevent deformities, in certain cases, by correctly positioning the joint.

Supports (sometimes called *braces*) are strong, elasticized wraps designed to fit certain body parts (your wrist, knee, ankle, and so on). Their tight fit lends stability to the joint, while their elasticity allows movement and blood circulation.

Supports are used two ways: to support and stabilize an injured joint or to protect a weakened joint from becoming injured in the first place. You should use supports in conjunction with a good exercise program, so the muscles and supporting structures themselves become strengthened and don't rely solely on the wrap to do the trick.

Magnets

Magnets seem to be everywhere these days. You can buy them at the local pharmacy, at medical supply stores, via mail-order houses, and even at the grocery store! Magnets used for pain relief are generally embedded within a belt or wrap designed to fit a specific body part (your neck, knee, ankle, wrist, and so on). You can also purchase them in sets that you can tape wherever the pain settles.

The magnets used for pain relief are much like the horseshoe-shaped toy you used to play with as a child, except they are small, flat discs. Just like your old toy, they exert a *pull* — a magnetic field that can attract or repel certain elements in the environment. A few researchers propose that this magnetic field can produce a calming effect on the body and help normalize bodily function. More important, the magnetic field helps block pain signals to the brain causing a release of endorphins, the body's own, natural morphine. Finally, like many of the other pain relieving techniques that we discuss in this chapter, magnets may help increase blood flow to the painful area.

You can gauge the power of a magnet by reading the label on the packaging, which lists a certain amount of *gauss*. Therapeutic magnets are measured in the hundreds or thousands of gauss. (By way of comparison, the earth's natural magnetic field is approximately .05 gauss and refrigerator magnets weigh in with about 60 gauss.) The actual amount of gauss delivered to the skin is much less than the amount listed, however. For example, a 6,000 gauss magnet may only transmit 1,800 gauss to the skin. And, the more wrapping or distance there is between the magnet and the skin, the weaker the magnetic effect. If possible, find a physical therapist or other health professional well-versed in magnetic therapy who can advise you.

Although the beneficial effects of magnets have been documented in at least one study, mainstream medicine has yet to fully embrace their use as a valid therapy. If you'd like to try magnetic therapy, consult with your doctor first. If you're pregnant or have a pacemaker or other electronic implant, you may not be a candidate for this treatment.

Transcutaneous electrical nerve stimulation (TENS)

Transcutaneous electrical nerve stimulation (TENS) is a mild electrical buzz that overrides pain signals in tender areas. The process may sound scary, but it really isn't, and it's easy to apply. Electrodes are affixed to your skin with a small amount of gel, and then a very mild shock (from a battery-powered unit connected to the electrodes) is transmitted to the pained area. As a result of these shocks, the production of endorphins is supposed to increase. The physiologic basis for TENS is the Gate Theory of Pain (discussed in Chapter 13). TENS helps to "close the gates," thus inhibiting pain impulses.

TENS is usually used to treat back and spine problems that don't respond to other treatments. It offers welcome temporary relief to many people, but it's not a cure.

You can purchase your own TENS unit and give yourself treatments at home, but only with a doctor's prescription. (If you decide to do your own treatments, learning to operate the TENS unit properly is important. Some people don't benefit from TENS simply because they use the equipment incorrectly.) Because the units are very expensive, you'll want to try TENS at your doctor's office several times before purchasing your own unit. Then, if you think it's worthwhile, you might consider renting one for awhile before committing yourself to a purchase.

Don't use TENS if you have a pacemaker or are pregnant. Also, don't use it on open wounds or sensitive parts of the body, such as the eyes.

Part III
The Arthritis Lifestyle Strategy

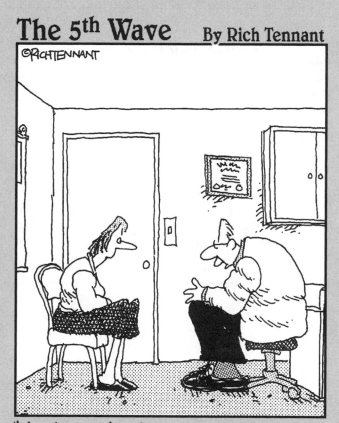

The 5th Wave   By Rich Tennant

"A change in diet can also help your arthritis. The next time you're at a restaurant, go ahead and order those bioflavonoids, and treat yourself to some Chondroitin sulfates..."

In this part . . .

*E*ven though arthritis is a medical problem that continues to baffle doctors, there's a great deal that you can
do at home to lessen your pain, improve your ability to
enjoy life and perform everyday tasks — and in some
cases, even slow the progression of the disease.

In this part, we tell you how to fight arthritis pain through
diet and supplements; how to keep your joints "loose" and
as mobile as possible through exercise; how walking,
sitting, and moving correctly can protect your joints; and
how to deal effectively with depression and anger. Plus,
you'll get loads of tips on how to make day-to-day living
with arthritis easier.

Chapter 10

Fighting the Pain with Foods and Supplements

*T*he idea that food can cause or relieve arthritis is not new. More than two hundred years ago, English doctors prescribed cod-liver oil to treat gout and rheumatism. More recently, some health writers have insisted that arthritics should eat or not eat specific foods. The debate is in full swing. Do certain foods cause arthritis? Is there an "Arthritis Begone" diet? All the evidence isn't yet in, but thanks to the studies currently available, more and more physicians are convinced that diet plays a valuable role in arthritis treatment plans.

And what about supplements? Can they eliminate arthritis pain, unlock "frozen" joints, or prevent the immune system errors that lead to rheumatoid arthritis? Researchers have not yet come up with definitive answers, but more and more scientific evidence suggests that supplements can be helpful aids in the battle against arthritis. So get ready and learn about some of the foods, "food parts," and supplements that can help and a few that might best be avoided.

Foods That Heal

Way back in the 1920s, researchers were looking into treating osteoarthritis with the mineral sulfur. In 1963, a letter to the editor in the prestigious medical journal called *Lancet* described the use of a B vitamin called pantothenic acid in treating osteoarthritis. The idea that foods and the vitamins, minerals, and other substances they contain can aid in the battle against arthritis is not new. What is new is that researchers are finding out why certain foods can be helpful — exactly why an apple a day may keep the doctor away.

Which fruits, vegetables, meat, or fish should you eat? There are no absolute rules, but the results of studies and case histories suggest that these foods may be helpful:

- **Anchovies:** Three-and-a-half ounces of anchovies contain almost a gram and a half of omega-3 fatty acids. The omega-3 fatty acids help regulate the prostaglandins, which play a role in inflammation and, hence, pain. However, anchovies are extremely high in sodium, so if sodium-sensitivity or water retention is a problem for you, choose a different kind of fish.

- **Apples:** Not only can an apple a day keep the doctor away, but it may also help to hold your arthritis at bay. Apples contain boron, a mineral that appears to reduce the risk of developing osteoarthritis. And when boron was given to people who already have the disease, it helped relieve pain.

- **Cantaloupe:** This sweet fruit contains large amounts of vitamin C and *beta-carotene,* the plant form of vitamin A. These two powerful vitamins help to control the oxidative and free-radical damage that may contribute to arthritis. (For more on oxidative and free-radical damage, see "Joint Saving Supplements" in this chapter.)

- **Chili peppers:** Chilies contain capsaicin, which gives them their heat. It also helps to block pain by encouraging certain nerve cells to run through their supply of substance P, which they normally use to help transmit pain signals.

- **Curry:** A combination of spices that often includes turmeric, garlic, cumin, cinnamon, and so on, curry contains powerful antioxidants that may help relieve inflammation and reduce pain.

- **Fish:** The omega-3 fatty acids in Norwegian sardines, Atlantic mackerel, sablefish, rainbow trout, striped bass, and other fish may help reduce inflammation and pain. (See "Using omega-3s and omega-6s to fight inflammation" in this chapter.)

- **Garlic:** An ancient treatment for tuberculosis, lung problems, and other diseases, garlic also appears to relieve some forms of arthritis pain. Although never tested in large-scale, double-blind studies, garlic has been found helpful in many case reports. These helpful benefits may be due to the fact that garlic contains sulfur, which has been known for many years to help relieve certain arthritis symptoms.

✔ **Grapes:** These bunches of sweet, bite-sized fruit are good sources of the mineral boron, which is important for strong bones.

✔ **Mango:** A sweet treat, mangoes are packed with three powerful antioxidants: 90 percent of the RDA (Recommended Dietary Allowances) for vitamin C, 75 percent of the daily dose of beta-carotene, plus vitamin E.

✔ **Nuts:** Almonds, peanuts, and hazelnuts are good sources of boron, a mineral that helps keep bones strong and certain arthritis symptoms at bay.

✔ **Papaya:** Long used as a folk medicine for diarrhea, hay fever, and other problems, a single papaya contains three times the RDA for the antioxidant vitamin C, plus more than half the daily allotment of beta-carotene.

✔ **Water:** Drinking eight glasses of water per day can help battle gout by flushing uric acid from the body. Eight glasses is also the amount most health experts recommend to keep your body moisturized and healthy.

Using omega-3s and omega-6s to fight inflammation

Fat is considered a boogey-man. It causes heart disease, and it contributes to obesity, cancer, and a host of other ills. You're told to cut the fat off of your meat and out of your diet. But certain kinds of fat, specifically the omega-3 and one type of omega-6 fatty acids, can be aids against arthritis.

Omega-3 fatty acids

Some interesting studies and case histories have suggested that omega-3 fatty acids may help relieve the pain and inflammation seen in some types of arthritis and related diseases. Strong evidence exists that omega-3 acids can help ease rheumatoid arthritis (RA) symptoms, help prevent Raynaud's spasms, and possibly relieve some lupus symptoms.

You can get omega-3 fatty acids from fish such as Chinook salmon and Atlantic mackerel. In general, the best sources of omega-3 fatty acids are fish that come from cold water. Fish from warmer waters and those raised on fish farms have less. You can also find omega-3 fatty acids in other foods, including butter nuts, black walnuts, and green soybeans.

What does "omega" mean?

A fatty acid is built around a line of carbon atoms. There may be a few, six, ten, twelve, or more carbons lined up, one behind the other, like a line of school children. Each of the carbons has a "left hand" and a "right hand," and can "hold" one hydrogen atom in each hand, off to either side. If each of the carbons in the line is holding two hydrogens, one in each hand, the fatty acid is saturated. Like a sponge that's full of water (saturated), the fatty acid can't possibly hold any more.

Often times, however, some of the carbons in the line "let go" of one of their hydrogens. Now

they're each holding only one. When that happens, the fatty acid is either unsaturated or polyunsaturated (depending on how many carbons have let go of a hydrogen).

If the first carbon holding only one hydrogen happens to be the third in line, the fatty acid is called an omega-3 fatty acid. If the first carbon holding only a single hydrogen is sixth in line, it's called an omega-6 fatty acid, and so on. They're called "omega" this or "omega" that because the counting starts at the side of the fatty acid called the omega side.

Likewise, you can get omega-3s through supplements. If you use a supplement, make sure that it clearly lists the amount of DHA and EPA per capsule. There is no RDA for fish oil: Some authorities suggest taking 3 grams of DHA and/or EPA per day.

Only take supplements after discussing them with your physician. And make sure you doctor always knows what supplements you are taking, for they may interfere with certain aspects of treatment.

Sources of omega-3 fatty acids

In general, the best sources of omega-3 fatty acids are fish that come from cold water. Fish from warmer waters and those raised on fish-farms have less.

Fish	Grams of omega-3 Per 3½ ounces raw fish
Roe	2.3
Atlantic mackerel	2.3
Pacific herring	1.6
Atlantic herring	1.5
Pacific mackerel	1.4
King salmon	1.3
Spanish mackerel	1.3
Pink salmon	1.0

You'll also find omega-3 fatty acids in other foods, including butter nuts, black walnuts, and green soybeans.

Omega-3 fatty acids have some long, complicated names such as *alpha-linolenic acid, DHA (docosahexaenoic acid),* and *EPA (eicosapentaenoic acid).* But, they're often referred to as omega-3s or fish oil, for short, because that's where you typically find them in their most concentrated form.

Taking fish oil and GLA (gamma linolenic acid) thins the blood, which can be dangerous if pushed too far. Overly thin blood may not clot properly, causing bleeding to increase to dangerous levels. Consult a physician before taking fish oil supplements if you take blood-thinning medication, NSAIDs, supplements that contain ginger, or anything else that thins the blood.

Don't deep-fry your fish. Doing so destroys the omega-3s.

The good omega-6 fatty acid — GLA

Although most of the omega-6s are best avoided (see the section on "Foods to Avoid," below), one of them gives hope to arthritis patients: gamma-linolenic acid, or GLA for short. Several studies have shown that GLA helps reduce pain and inflammation in RA patients, and it may also help with other forms of arthritis.

You won't find large amounts of GLA in food. Besides evening primrose oil, good sources of GLA include borage oil and black currant oil. An often-suggested dose is 1 to 2 grams of GLA per day. Make sure that the primrose oil or other product you purchase lists the GLA content on the label so you know exactly how many capsules or spoonfuls you need to take to get the desired dosage. You can purchase evening primrose oil, borage oil, and black currant oil in health food stores.

Foods to Avoid

No foods actually *cause* arthritis. At worst, they may exacerbate a preexisting condition. For example, alcohol can trigger gout, but only in certain people. However, there are foods that give some people trouble, so you may want to consider cutting back or avoiding intake of the following:

- ✔ **Nightshades:** Peppers, potatoes, eggplant, and tomatoes are some of the members of the nightshade family of vegetables. Some people feel that eating nightshades aggravates their rheumatoid arthritis and other forms of the disease. Although this hasn't been proven, if you feel that eating nightshades worsens your symptoms, avoid them.

✓ **Organ meats:** Liver, kidney, sweet bread, and other organ meats contain the purines that can trigger gout. If you have gout, avoid organ meat and other foods high in purines, including sardines, anchovies, and meat gravies.

✓ **Processed meat:** Cold cuts, hot dogs, bacon, and other processed meats contain various chemicals that may trigger allergic reactions, bringing about arthritis-like symptoms. Or, they may cause flare-ups of existing arthritis conditions. It's not clear whether these substances actually trigger arthritis or allergies, or whether they tend to replace the vegetables, fruits, and whole grains that provide nutrients needed to hold arthritis at bay.

✓ **Foods containing linoleic/arachidonic acid:** The omega-3 fatty acids help reduce inflammation, but linoleic acid, an omega-6 fatty acid, does the opposite. Linoleic acid is found in salad or cooking oils, such as corn, safflower, and sunflower. It's used to make many kinds of fast food, and large amounts of it are fed to the cattle that eventually end up in the meat department of your grocery store. Linoleic acid is converted into arachidonic acid, which the body uses to build the substances that trigger inflammation and arthritic pain. Naturally, the less linoleic acid you consume, the better for your arthritis! To avoid linoleic acid, switch to olive, flaxseed, or canola oil for cooking, eat less meat and poultry, and avoid fast foods. At the same time, increase your consumption of the fish and other foods that contain the helpful omega-3 fatty acids (see "Omega-3 fatty acids," earlier in this section).

Watch for food allergies

If you've noticed that a food tends to make your arthritis worse, try eliminating it from your diet for awhile to see if doing so helps. There are many reports (including some published in prestigious medical journals) of arthritis cases being "cured" when the sufferer stopped eating certain foods, including cheese, corn, milk, and various members of the nightshade vegetable family. Most likely, their arthritis-like symptoms were the result of simple food allergies. This diagnosis may not be true for you, but it's certainly worth a try.

To test for a food allergy, eliminate all foods that contain the suspected culprit for at least two weeks and keep a diary so that you can write down everything you eat and drink, plus your symptoms — especially any reactions or changes in the way you feel. After the two-week period, if you've noticed no difference, gradually add the foods back into your diet, one at a time, in small amounts, once again recording your diet, symptoms, and any changes. Remember: This test is not a true, scientifically valid elimination diet. Only a health professional can conduct a scientifically valid elimination diet.

Joint-Saving Supplements

Various studies have linked poor nutrition to rheumatoid arthritis, juvenile arthritis, and other forms of the disease. However, the connection between nutrition and arthritis isn't yet fully understood. For example, researchers can't say that eating too few apples will cause arthritis, or that drinking too much beer *always* triggers gout. However, it's clear that good nutrition is an important part of the battle against arthritis. Evidence also suggests that careful use of supplements can be very helpful. And it's not just the omega-3 and omega-6 fatty acids that can help. Antioxidants and free radical scavengers, plus some regular vitamins and minerals, can also have beneficial effects.

Take *all* supplements with care, because even helpful ones can interact with medicines or herbs that you're taking and cause trouble. Supplements can increase the effectiveness of blood-thinning medications, making you more likely to bleed unnecessarily; counteract the effectiveness of some immune system-suppressing drugs; increase the side effects of NSAIDs; make alcohol and sedatives more powerful; hinder the absorption of select nutrients; and so on. It's always best to let your physician know about *all* the supplements, herbs, and other substances you are taking. Consult with him or her before beginning to take supplements, increasing or decreasing the dosage, or discontinuing their use.

What oxidants and free radicals do

Here's a short list of the damage that oxidants and/or free radicals can do:

✔ They can attack the fatty membranes surrounding body cells. With repeated hits, the cell membrane may eventually become damaged, unable to ferry water, oxygen, and nutrients into the cells and waste products out. In short, the cell will be unable to function properly.

✔ Sometimes they can harm the outer wall of the cell, and parts of the cell will leak out. In the wake of the spill, neighboring cells can be damaged.

✔ They can severely damage the DNA that makes up the genetic blueprints within your cells. When this happens, your cells may be unable to grow, function and/or repair themselves properly.

✔ They can increase the inflammation response. (The inflammation response is the body's answer to foreign invaders, such as bacteria, and to injury. During the inflammation response, fluid rushes to the afflicted area, and the immune system is mo-bilized. Inflammation is a by-product of the immune system's attempt to destroy the foreign invader or repair the damage.)

✔ They can hamper the immune system, the same internal defense system that goes awry in some forms of arthritis. (The immune system sometimes uses oxidants and free radicals to fight off certain germs. But these same "weapons" can harm the immune system: it's like a soldier being shot with his own gun.)

Oxidants and free radicals

Oxidants and free radicals are perfectly normal substances in the body; they're the result of normal metabolism. Unfortunately, if not properly controlled by the body, they can cause damage to cells, tissues, and organs, and have been linked to many ailments, including arthritis. Researchers can't absolutely say that they *cause* arthritis, but they're implicated in actions that lay the groundwork for trouble — or make current trouble worse.

Fortunately, there are many oxidant-quenching and free radical–corralling substances called *antioxidants* and *free radical quenchers* in foods and supplements. These may help you fight the cellular damage that can contribute to arthritis.

Vitamin C

This popular vitamin works together with vitamin E to scavenge free radicals or stabilize them so they're no longer dangerous. It also helps reactivate used vitamin E so it can charge back into the fray. In the late 1990s, researchers reported that vitamin C may also help halt the progression of osteoarthritis.

Fresh fruits and vegetables, especially papaya, guava, red peppers, cantaloupe, sweet green peppers, oranges, broccoli, cauliflower, and asparagus are good sources of vitamin C. An often-suggested dose is 500 mg of vitamin C or more per day in supplement form.

Vitamin E

Vitamin E helps fight arthritis in at least two ways. First, just like NSAIDs, it slows the action of the prostaglandins that play a major role in producing pain. Second, it helps control the free radicals that can damage cells and tissues in and around the joint. There have also been individual reports suggesting that vitamin E may help in the treatment of Raynaud's.

Vitamin E is found in a variety of foods, including green leafy vegetables, broccoli, brussels sprouts, seeds, nuts, green beans, and wheat germ oil. An often-suggested dose is 400 to 600 IU per day in supplement form.

Selenium

Selenium, an essential mineral with antioxidant properties, works together with *glutathione peroxidase* (one of the body's internal defenders) to control free radicals. Selenium also makes vitamin E more effective.

You find selenium in whole grains, fish, poultry, and meat; smaller amounts are present in fruits and vegetables. Selenium levels in food vary, depending in part on how much of the mineral was in the ground where the food was grown. An often-suggested dose is 100 to 200 mg per day in supplement form.

Boron: Strong bones and osteoarthritis

The vital mineral boron doesn't get much respect from the public — mostly because the public's not familiar with it. But boron helps regulate calcium (a mineral key to bone health), keeping it from leaving the bones and the body. Although boron's role in arthritis isn't completely clear, it can help relieve inflammation and appears to be helpful in combating both osteoarthritis and rheumatoid arthritis.

Boron is found in a variety of foods, including apples, peaches, peas, beans, lentils, peanuts, almonds, and grapes. An often-suggested dose is 1 to 2 mg or more per day in supplement form.

Vitamin B₆: Relieves carpal tunnel

Vitamin B_6, also known as *pyridoxine,* assists the body in making hormones, hemoglobin, neurotransmitters, and many of the enzymes necessary for life. This vitamin also helps to relieve the pain and stiffness of carpal tunnel syndrome and, in some cases, can make surgery unnecessary.

You find vitamin B_6 in brewer's yeast, sunflower seeds, wheat germ, soybeans, walnuts, lentils, black-eyed peas, navy beans, bananas, brown rice, and many other foods. An often-suggested dose is 50 mg or more per day in supplement form.

Niacin combats Raynaud's

Niacin is a member of the B-vitamin family. It was first noted early in the twentieth century during the battle against *pellagra,* the disease that causes blotchy skin rashes, confusion, weakness, memory loss, and other problems. Pellagra is rarely seen today, and doctors are primarily interested in niacin's ability to keep the skin, nerves, and intestines healthy, to lower cholesterol, and possibly guard against cancer.

Niacin also has some antirheumatic properties. For example, Raynaud's patients given a niacin preparation reported fewer and shorter attacks of the disease as compared to Raynaud's patients given a placebo. Nuts, liver, fortified grains and cereals, peanut butter, milk, cheese, and fish are good sources of niacin. An often-suggested dose is 10 to 15 mg or more per day in supplement form. Niacin should be taken in the form of niacinamide to minimize side effects (for example, severe facial flushing).

Zinc: Rheumatoid and psoriatic arthritis

The mineral zinc is necessary for many aspects of good health. Although no one has shown that a lack of zinc causes arthritis, researchers know that the amount of zinc in the blood is lower than it should be in at least some people suffering from rheumatoid arthritis, which suggests that zinc supplements may help some rheumatic arthritis patients.

The results of studies with zinc on arthritis have been mixed. Some have shown that zinc helps, others have shown that it has no significant benefit. This has led some researchers to suggest that zinc may not be helpful for everyone, but can be a great aid to carefully selected arthritis patients who have low levels of the mineral.

The jury is still out on zinc. It may help, and hundreds of thousands of people take it every day without suffering harmful side effects. Many researchers feel that zinc will help *certain* people; the key is to figure out exactly whom.

You can find zinc in oysters, seafood, eggs, meat, wheat germ, and plain yogurt. An often-suggested dose is 50 mg per day in supplement form.

Other Substances for Relieving Arthritis Symptoms

Omega-3 fatty acids, GLA (the "good" omega-6 fatty acid), antioxidants, free radical quenchers, vitamins, and minerals: The nutritional arsenal against arthritis is growing larger every year. And there's more. Here are a few of the nonvitamin, nonmineral, nonantioxidant substances that are gaining recognition.

Aloe vera

Made from the leaves of the aloe plant, aloe vera juice is an ancient beauty aid, reportedly used by Cleopatra to keep her skin fresh and soft. It is also an all-purpose balm that was carried by Alexander the Great's soldiers as they conquered much of the ancient world. Today, aloe vera juice's popularity is partially due to its inflammation-relieving properties. Many people drink aloe juice as a laxative and health-booster, and aloe vera creams or gels are used to treat sunburn, cuts, burns, and abrasions. Stabilized aloe vera juice contains numerous vitamins, minerals, and amino acids, which may explain its many beneficial effects.

There are reports that drinking aloe juice can help relieve symptoms of rheumatoid arthritis as well as other inflammatory forms of arthritis. A few animal studies back up these claims, and many arthritis sufferers are eagerly awaiting human studies that will show that aloe can help knock down arthritis symptoms. Meanwhile, many people insist that moderate amounts of aloe juice relieve swelling.

You can find aloe vera in juice, cream, gel, and capsule form. An often-suggested dose is up to 200 mg or more per day in capsule form.

SAMe

Gaining fame as a remedy for heart disease, depression, and other ailments, SAMe (short for S-adenosyl-L-methione and pronounced *sammy*) is naturally produced by the body. In turn, SAMe helps the body manufacture a vital hormone called melatonin, which plays an important role in the sleep process. SAMe also protects DNA.

Since at least the late 1980s, SAMe has also strutted its stuff as a painkiller that's particularly effective in osteoarthritis. When placed head-to-head against four standard arthritis medicines (ibuprofen, indomethacin, piroxicam, and naproxen), SAMe proved to be just as effective — with fewer side effects than some of these drugs. It's also been shown to counteract depression as well as a standard antidepressant, with few side effects. The supplement has been used to treat osteoarthritis in Europe for many years.

As often-suggested dose is up to 400 mg per day in divided doses, three times a day, as a supplement. SAMe is available without a prescription in many health food and vitamin stores.

Capsaicin

Chili peppers have long been used to treat numerous ills, including (surprisingly enough) indigestion! Today, researchers know that the *capsaicin,* the ingredient that gives chilies their bite, can help relieve pain.

Creams containing capsaicin are available in many drugstores without a prescription. Apply the cream to the painful area, following the instructions on the label.

Some people find capsaicin irritating, so if you decide to try it, start with a very small trial dose and work your way up.

Grapeseed extract

Medical researchers haven't yet discovered all the ins and outs of grapeseed extract, but it appears to help vitamin C cross into certain body cells. With a good supply of vitamin C safely tucked inside, these cells are better able to prevent and/or repair oxidative damage. Grapeseed also helps combat the inflammation associated with many forms of arthritis by slowing the body's release of enzymes that increase inflammation.

Grapeseed extract is available as a supplement. An often-suggested dose is 60 mg per day in supplement form.

Flaxseed oil

Many people swear by flaxseed oil, which contains many "parts" that the body can turn into the helpful omega-3 fatty acid known as EPA. A few studies look promising, and many reports suggest that flaxseed oil can help reduce the inflammation of rheumatoid and possibly other forms of arthritis.

Flaxseed comes in oil or capsule form and as flour or a meal. You can use the oil for cooking or as a topping, bake with the flour or meal, and sprinkle the seeds on cereals and other foods. An often-suggested daily dose is a few tablespoons of the oil, the equivalent in capsule form, or up to a third cup of the flour or meal.

Glucosamine sulfate and chondroitin sulfate: Cures for osteoarthritis?

In early 1997, two supplements burst upon the arthritis scene: glucosamine and chondroitin sulfate. Although touted as new, veterinarians had used them for years to relieve arthritis or arthritis-like symptoms in horses and other animals.

Unlike standard drugs for osteoarthritis, which are designed to relieve symptoms, glucosamine and chondroitin appear to help the body (specifically the cartilage) heal itself. Together, glucosamine and chondroitin increase production of *collagen*, the framework of cartilage; slow certain enzymes that prematurely destroy cartilage; block enzymes that interfere with the transfer of nutrients to the cartilage; and increase the production of proteoglycans, the molecules that help keep cartilage wet and healthy.

Pulling together the results from many studies using either or both of these two supplements gives a promising picture. Here are some of the exciting results:

- ✔ Osteoarthritis patients reported that their pain levels dropped, often significantly.

- ✔ Patients who had difficulty walking were now able to increase the rate at which they walked a measured distance by 30 percent or more.

- ✔ Symptoms such as pain sometimes disappeared altogether.

- ✔ Erosion of the cartilage was sometimes slowed or halted.

- ✔ Study participants experienced few or no side effects.

- ✔ People taking glucosamine and chondroitin sulfate were often able to reduce their NSAID dosage.

- ✔ The positive benefits did not fade with time, unlike the benefits reaped from many other medicines.

- ✔ The medicinal effect continued even after patients stopped taking the supplements.

- ✔ The two supplements were as effective as ibuprofen, an often-prescribed NSAID, but were better tolerated because they lacked the side effects typically seen with drugs.

Not everyone will experience all the positive benefits of these two substances, of course, and researchers don't yet know who is most likely to benefit. Glucosamine and chondroitin are not fast-acting, like pain pills, so you can expect to wait anywhere from a few days to several weeks before you feel the difference. If you don't notice any improvement within a few months, it's a good bet that the two supplements aren't for you.

There are many different brands of glucosamine and chondroitin sulfate supplements. An often-suggested dose is 1,000 to 2,000 mg of glucosamine and 800 to 1,200 mg of chondroitin sulfate.

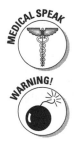

There are several forms of glucosamine, including glucosamine sulfate, glucosamine hydrochloride and n-acetyl glucosamine. Although most of the studies have been conducted with the sulfate form, the hydrochloride form is believed to be just as effective. Some researchers feel that the n-acetyl form is weaker than the other two.

If you're allergic to sulfates, avoid glucosamine sulfate and chondroitin sulfate.

DPLA's history

Almost 30 years ago, researchers at the Johns Hopkins University School of Medicine were startled to find that the human brain manufactured substances surprisingly similar to morphine. Dubbing the newly discovered substances *endorphins*, which means "morphine within," the researchers began to investigate. They quickly learned that one endorphin, *beta-endorphin*, was 18 to 50 times more powerful than morphine, the most powerful painkiller known. Another endorphin, called *dynorphin*, was even stronger!

The discovery of endorphins was thrilling, but it made scientists wonder: Why did the human body make these very powerful painkillers? The answer, they decided, was that they were designed to be part of the human body's natural, built-in pain-relief system. This made sense, but brought up another question: If we have a built-in pain relief system, why do many of us hurt so much?

The answer to this question is fairly simple: Although the body is making endorphins, it's also making "endorphin-eaters" to keep these powerful painkillers in line, for too many endorphins can be as dangerous as too few. After all, you need to feel pain sometimes in order to avoid injuring yourself. But in cases of chronic pain, scientists theorize, the endorphin-eaters gain the upper hand and destroy endorphins faster than they can be produced. The result is a lack of the natural pain-killers and, of course, more pain.

This discovery set the scientists on a quest to discover an endorphin shield — a way to protect endorphins from being destroyed before their time so they can continue to kill our pain.

In no time at all, the endorphin shield was discovered — a modest, unassuming amino acid called *phenylalanine* (fennel-al-a-neen). More specifically, it was a form called *dl-phenylalanine*, or DLPA. *DLPA* guards the endorphins against early destruction, allowing endorphin levels to rise so they can block the pain.

DLPA (dl-phenylalanine)

Studies have confirmed that DLPA is a natural, safe, and effective means of controlling arthritis pain in many people. Studies have shown that DLPA is safer than standard arthritis drugs and, in the long run, costs less. It takes longer to take effect than aspirin or other NSAIDs, but the relief lasts longer. And, because it improves body chemistry, DLPA continues working for days and sometimes even weeks after you stop using it.

Because DLPA is an amino acid (a natural food substance), you can purchase it in health food and vitamin stores. An often-suggested dose is 300 to 400 mg per day, three times a day (with breakfast, lunch, and dinner).

Consult your physician before taking this supplement. If you suffer from the genetic disease phenylketonuria (PKU), or if you're on a phenylalanine-restricted diet, you shouldn't take DLPA. Likewise, children, pregnant, or lactating women shouldn't take DLPA.

Looking at a Possible Link between Lupus and Food

There are no easy nutritional answers for *lupus,* one of the more puzzling and complex forms of rheumatic disease. Studies with mice suggest that a low-calorie, low-fat diet may help improve the symptoms, possibly by reducing abnormal immune system responses.

Certain vitamins may also be helpful adjuncts to lupus treatment. For example:

- ✔ Intravenous injections of niacin improved (but did not eliminate) skin lesions in systemic lupus patients.
- ✔ Pantothenic acid given in large doses caused improvement in patients with systemic and discoid lupus.
- ✔ Injecting vitamin B_{12} into three patients who had systemic lupus cleared up their skin lesions in six weeks.
- ✔ Vitamin E eased the symptoms in 9 out of 12 people with systemic lupus.
- ✔ Within one to six months, 67 people enjoyed improvement in their symptoms when given daily doses of pantothenic acid plus vitamin E.

Taking a detailed look at all the supplements that people take for their various forms of arthritis is beyond the scope of this book, but this brief account will give you enough information to start a discussion with your doctor. In fact, this is a key point: Discuss *everything* you plan to take with your physician. There are subtle and sometimes hidden reactions caused by the combination of body chemistry, supplements, medications, and disease processes that may make your situation worse.

Chapter 11

Oiling Your Joints with Exercise

In This Chapter

▶ Fighting arthritis with exercise

▶ Improving endurance

▶ Building strength

▶ Increasing flexibility and range of motion

▶ Designing your own fitness plan

*A*t our local gym there's a sign that says "Warning: Not Exercising is Hazardous to Your Health!" This truth goes double for arthritis sufferers, because a lack of exercise can do a number on your joints, making them stiffer, less mobile, and more likely to degenerate. The old saying, "Use it or lose it!" is an appropriate one for those who live with arthritis. In this chapter, we discuss the elements of a good fitness program and give you tips on setting up a plan that can help strengthen your joints without disrupting your lifestyle.

Before you start on any kind of exercise program, consult your physician to determine whether your body can accommodate the stresses of exercise. This is especially critical if you haven't exercised in awhile, if you're over 40, or you have heart disease or high blood pressure.

Different Exercises for Different Goals

Every good fitness plan, no matter how simple or complex, includes three basic kinds of exercise: *cardiovascular endurance*, *strength training* and *flexibility*. Together, these three types of exercise can build a strong, toned and healthy body that's more able to withstand physical, mental, and emotional stresses. Your initial goal should be to follow a short, easy fitness plan that includes these three kinds of exercise. Then you can slowly increase the length and intensity of the exercises as you become more physically fit.

A physical therapist or exercise physiologist experienced in working with people who have arthritis should design and supervise your fitness program. Any kind of exercise, whether cardiovascular endurance, strength training, or flexibility, can cause injury if done improperly, especially over time.

Cardiovascular endurance exercises

Countless studies have shown that people who do cardiovascular endurance exercises regularly have less heart disease, more energy, less body fat, lower blood pressure and cholesterol levels, faster metabolisms, higher self-esteem, and a greater sense of well-being. After you've warmed up with some moderately-paced walking or calisthenics, you can safely move on to these exercises that rev up your body's motor. You'll have to become a heavy breather, however, because cardiovascular endurance exercises that are done properly make your breath come faster and your heart beat more quickly.

There's a host of invigorating activities from which you can choose: walking, swimming, cycling, ballroom dancing, and so on. If you enjoy the outdoors, try a brisk walk or hike. If you prefer climate-controlled conditions, why not dance or ride a stationary bike? You can also try a water aerobics class held in a heated pool.

Take advantage of the great variety of fun and exciting cardio-endurance exercises available, and mix them up in your individual fitness plan. For example, you may swim during one session, ride a bike in the next, and take a jitterbug class in the third. It's important to do different kinds of exercise that work out different parts of your body so that you'll increase overall fitness and not put too much stress on any one area.

Strength training

Strength training exercises improve the ability of your muscles to do work by increasing the force they can exert *(strength)* and the length of time that they can exert that force *(endurance)*. If you have arthritis, strength training is particularly important because strong, well-toned muscles and other supporting structures can help absorb the stress and strain placed on your joints. Weak muscles do just the opposite, forcing your joints to bear the brunt of impact, and encouraging joint misalignment or slippage. Your weight-bearing joints (those in your spine, hips, knees and ankles) and their supporting structures (tendons, ligaments, muscles and so on) also need to be sturdy and strong enough to take on an additional load as your body tries to protect the injured or diseased area by shifting the weight elsewhere.

Weight and reps are the basis of strength training. You can build your strength by gradually increasing the amount of weight that your muscles must lift, which will make your muscles bigger and bulkier. But by increasing the number of times your muscles perform a certain movement (repetitions or reps), you can increase your endurance, which is even more important. Bulkier muscles are less flexible, more likely to be injured, and less likely to improve joint range of motion than muscles that have been conditioned for endurance.

Don't be fooled into believing that you can only do strength training with a set of barbells. When a dancer slowly lifts her leg and holds it in position, she is lifting weight — the weight of her leg as gravity pulls against it. When a swimmer pulls his arms through the water, he is working against the resistance of the water. With exercises like dancing and swimming, you don't need additional weights!

You can do different strength-enhancing exercises to vary your workouts and keep your exercise plan fresh and interesting while toning different muscle groups. Strength-enhancing exercises include the following:

- Isometric exercises
- Sit-ups
- Push-ups
- Leg lifts
- Weight training
- Swimming
- Stair climbing
- Cross-country skiing
- Dance or yoga (sustained poses)
- Running

There are two kinds of strength training exercises – *isotonic* and *isometric*. When performing *isotonic* exercises, your muscles move against the resistance of gravity, water, light weights, or your own body weight, and your joints bend and straighten. Weight lifting or swimming are two examples.

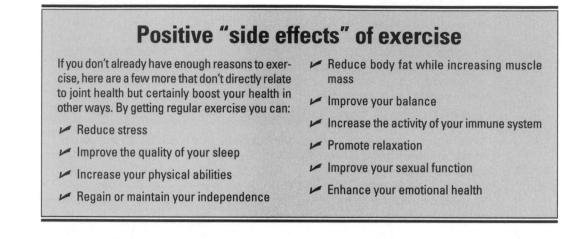

Positive "side effects" of exercise

If you don't already have enough reasons to exercise, here are a few more that don't directly relate to joint health but certainly boost your health in other ways. By getting regular exercise you can:

✔ Reduce stress

✔ Improve the quality of your sleep

✔ Increase your physical abilities

✔ Regain or maintain your independence

✔ Reduce body fat while increasing muscle mass

✔ Improve your balance

✔ Increase the activity of your immune system

✔ Promote relaxation

✔ Improve your sexual function

✔ Enhance your emotional health

Isometric exercises, on the other hand, are done *without* moving your joints. Muscles are contracted and released, but the joint stays in a static position. Often, your body itself provides the resistance. For example, clasping your hands in front of you and pushing them together is an isometric exercise for your arms and pectoral muscles. These exercises are great for toning your muscles and supporting structures on days when your joints are just too painful to move.

Flexibility

Flexibility exercises (stretching) increase your ability to bend, reach, twist, and stretch. They help you maintain or increase your *range of motion* — the amount of movement your joints allow in various directions. Flexibility exercises also improve the elasticity of your muscles, which makes them more resistant to injury. If you have arthritis, flexibility exercises are crucial, because pain, stiffness, and restricted range of motion tend to make you want to move your joints less, which only increases the pain, stiffness, and limited movement over time.

You may think that you already bend and stretch enough while doing housework or gardening, and that you can just skip flexibility exercises. But, everyday activities don't move your joints through their full range of motion, so you need to make flexibility exercises a regular part of your daily program. Try to do them every day if possible.

Exercises to Ease Joint Pain

There are countless exercises that can help make you stronger, more fit, more flexible, and better able to fight arthritis. Those that you choose will depend upon what you and your physical therapist feel are the best ones for your particular condition. Having said that, we include the exercises outlined below as good ones for stretching and/or strengthening the indicated areas.

For some of the exercises in this section, you need to use an exercise mat to protect your weight-bearing joints from excessive pressure when they're in contact with the floor.

Neck stretch

Use this exercise to stretch and relieve tension in your neck muscles:

1. Sit cross-legged on your exercise mat, hands resting comfortably on your knees or thighs. While facing to the front, drop your head to the right side, as if trying to touch your right ear to your right shoulder. (Don't scrunch up your shoulders!)

2. Put your right hand over the top of your head, and your left hand on top of your left shoulder.

3. Exert a gentle pressure with each hand, stretching your neck.

4. Repeat on the other side.

Hand and wrist stretches

This stretches and strengthens your fingers and wrists:

1. Make a fist.

2. Fling your fingers out to their straightened position, fingers spread.

3. Return to the fist position.

4. Repeat five times for each hand.

The following exercise increases finger and hand flexibility:

1. Open your hand flat.

2. Touch the tip of your thumb to the tip of each of your fingers, one at a time.

Shoulder arm extension

Use this exercise to strengthen your upper back and shoulder muscles:

1. Assume a hands-and-knees position on your exercise mat, with your neck straight and parallel to the floor.

2. Slowly reach your right arm out in front of you, keeping your arm straight, parallel to the floor and about the height of your ear. (Your fingers should point at the wall on the opposite side of the room.)

3. Hold for 5 seconds, if possible, and then slowly return your arm to its starting position.

4. Repeat with your other arm, and then alternate, doing as many reps as you can manage. (See Figure 11-1.)

Figure 11-1:
Shoulder arm extension. You'll need this in your upper back, but it can really help improve your posture.

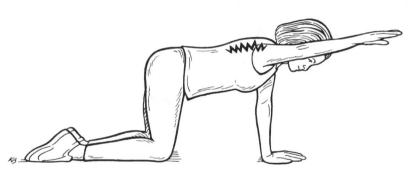

Side stretch

This exercise tones your side and back muscles and helps prevent sudden back spasms that can result from turning or twisting the wrong way.

1. Stand straight with your feet about 18 inches apart.

2. Bend your left elbow, placing your left hand at your waist.

3. Straighten your right arm above your head, while trying to keep your right shoulder level with the left one.

4. Bend slowly toward the left (toward your bent elbow), keeping your right arm above your head. You should feel a pull in your right side. Hold this position for a count of five. (Be careful not to push your right hip to the side as your bend — that's cheating and it can put stress on your knees.)

5. Slowly return to an upright position.

6. Repeat on the other side. (See Figure 11-2.)

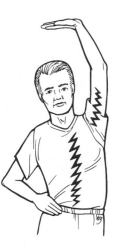

Lower back pelvic lift

This exercise tightens your rear-end muscles and stretches your lower back.

1. Lie on your back on your exercise mat, knees bent and a couple of inches apart, with the soles of your feet flat on the mat. Your arms should be straight and about 3 inches away from your sides, with your palms flat against the mat.

2. Tighten your buttock muscles and slowly raise your pelvis, supporting your weight with your feet and your lower arms. (Try to keep your spine straight — don't arch up — but don't let your rear-end sag, either. You should have a nice straight line from your shoulders to your knees.)

3. Hold this raised position for five seconds.

4. Slowly ease your back down, vertebrae by vertebrae, beginning with your upper back and ending with your tailbone.

5. Repeat slowly at least 5 times. (See Figure 11-3.)

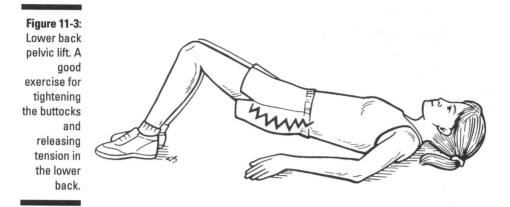

Figure 11-3: Lower back pelvic lift. A good exercise for tightening the buttocks and releasing tension in the lower back.

Hamstring stretch

Use this stretch to help you loosen up your lower back and back of your thighs (hamstrings), as well as to improve your ability to bend over.

1. Lie on your back on your exercise mat with your knees flexed and arms at your sides.

2. Bend your right knee and grab the back of your thigh with both hands.

3. Pull your knee toward your chest, keeping your foot pointed rather than flexed. (Flexing will stretch the sciatic nerve.)

4. While holding onto your thigh, extend the lower part of your leg until your leg is completely straight. If you can't straighten it, lower your leg until you can. Hold for a count of five.

5. Bend your knee and move your leg back to the mat.

6. Repeat with the other leg. (See Figure 11-4.)

If your arms aren't long enough to hold your leg while it's straightening, slide a towel or a belt around the back of your thigh and hold on to the ends of it. To benefit from this exercise, you need to keep your working leg as straight as possible, your supporting leg bent, and your back flat on the ground.

Mini sit-up

This exercise is great for tightening the abdominal muscles, which support your lower back. The mini sit-up causes your abdominals to contract and hold at the point of maximum resistance, without putting too much strain on your back and neck muscles.

1. Lying flat on your back on your exercise mat, bend your knees, keeping your feet flat on the floor. Your knees shouldn't be more than an inch or two apart.

2. Fold your arms across your chest and raise your head, neck, and shoulders off the floor. Your head and neck will curl forward, but they shouldn't curl so far forward that your chin is on your chest.

3. Hold this position for a count of five. Try not to let your stomach muscles pop out; instead, suck them in.

4. Slowly release and roll back down to your starting position.

5. Repeat this exercise five times, if possible. (See Figure 11-5.)

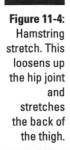

If you can't get your shoulders completely off the floor at first, don't worry. Do the best you can and work toward that goal in the long run.

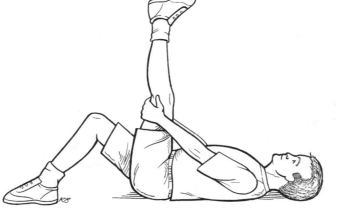

Figure 11-4:
Hamstring stretch. This loosens up the hip joint and stretches the back of the thigh.

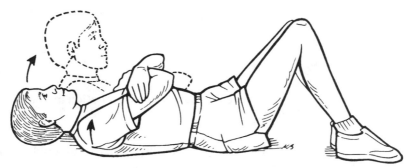

Figure 11-5:
Mini sit-up. This tightens the abdominal muscles without putting a lot of stress and strain on the back and neck.

Hip back leg extension

The buttock muscles are important in maintaining good posture. When they are contracted and "tucked under," the stomach muscles automatically contract, too. This helps you support your lower back, while avoiding the sway back, stomach out, knees locked position that is so detrimental to your joints. Use this exercise to tighten up your rear-end muscles:

1. Assume a hands-and-knees position on your exercise mat with your neck parallel to the floor.

2. When you feel comfortable and balanced, flex the toes of your right foot.

3. Slide your right leg out behind you until it's straight and supported only by your toes.

4. Slowly lift your right leg up until it's parallel with the floor.

5. Hold the position for 5 seconds.

6. Lower your leg slowly, bend it, and bring it back to its original position.

7. Repeat exercise with your left leg. (See Figure 11-6.)

Figure 11-6:
Hip back leg extension. This exercise helps support your lower back by stregthening the buttock muscles.

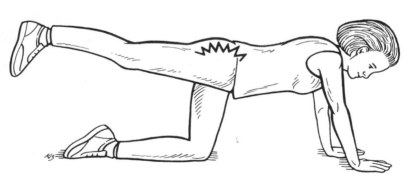

Ankle rotation

This exercise is great for increasing the range of motion in your ankle.

1. Lie on your back on your exercise mat, legs bent and arms at your sides.

2. Raise your right leg into the air, keeping it bent, and hold on to your right thigh for support.

3. Rotate your foot slowly in a circle to the right, as if drawing a circle in the air with your big toe.

4. Rotate four times to the right and four times to the left. Repeat the exercise with your left foot.

Using Yoga to Ease Arthritis Pain

Yoga, a branch of Ayurvedic healing, is an ancient way of bringing your physical, mental and spiritual "selves" into balance and harmony, thus achieving the highest form of good health. There are many kinds of yoga, but all involve assuming various sitting, standing or lying-down postures called *asanas*. The postures are held for anywhere from seconds to minutes and are accompanied by deep breathing.

The benefits of yoga for arthritis sufferers are many, including relaxation, stress reduction, increased energy, improved flexibility, increased strength, and improved circulation. As an added bonus, many people find that regularly practicing yoga helps relieve depression, increase alertness and improve overall well-being.

Don't try to learn yoga on your own by watching a videotape or reading a book. Instead, find a qualified instructor who has worked with people who have arthritis. Then, ease into yoga slowly — there's no rush — but practicing daily is recommended.

The snake

Use this posture, or *asana*, to stretch your chest, stomach, and upper back muscles while strengthening your arms and upper body.

1. On your exercise mat, lie face down on your stomach with your arms bent, hands palm down resting on either side of your neck.

2. Pressing your hands and lower arms into the mat, slowly raise your head and upper chest until they are completely off the floor.

3. Gradually straighten your arms as you push your head, chest, and torso as far up as you can. (Be sure to keep your pelvis flat on the floor and your legs extended.)

4. Hold position for a count of five.

5. Slowly bend your arms as you ease your torso down to the mat.

6. Gradually return to the starting position with your face on the mat. (See Figure 11-7.)

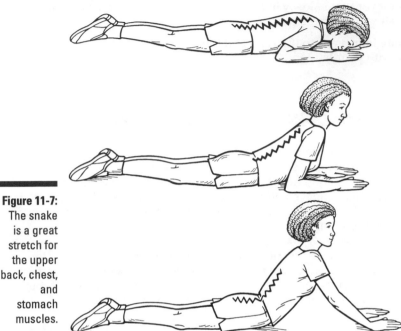

Figure 11-7:
The snake is a great stretch for the upper back, chest, and stomach muscles.

The cat

This exercise helps increase spinal flexibility.

1. Assume the hands-and-knees position on your exercise mat with your neck parallel to the floor. Your knees should be about 12 inches apart, with your arms straight down and your fingers pointing forward.

2. Contract your stomach muscles and roll your head forward until your chin touches your chest as you round your back upward toward the ceiling. Your entire torso should be contracted and forming a hollow.

3. Gradually release the contraction and roll your head back to its original position.

4. Arch your back slightly, creating a curve going the opposite way. (Don't stick your rear-end out, let your stomach muscles relax or sway your back to accomplish this position; these things can put too much pressure on the disks between your vertebrae.)

5. Repeat, slowly forming the hump, and then ease into a slight arch. (See Figure 11-8.)

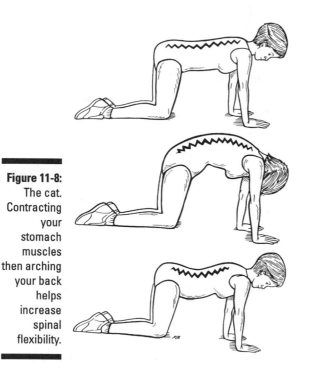

Figure 11-8:
The cat. Contracting your stomach muscles then arching your back helps increase spinal flexibility.

The pretzel

Use this exercise to stretch your inner thigh and hip.

1. Lie on your back on your exercise mat, legs bent and arms at your sides.

2. Cross your right leg over your left leg, with your right foot just clearing your left knee.

3. Grab your left thigh with both hands and pull it toward you while keeping your legs in the crossed position.

4. Hold this position for at least 5 seconds.

5. Slowly release, and then repeat with the opposite leg. (See Figure 11-9.)

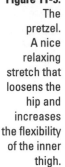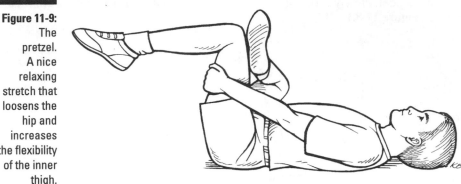

Knee to chest stretch

This exercise loosens up the hip joint while stretching your lower back and buttock muscles.

1. Lie on your back on your exercise mat, legs extended and arms at your sides.

2. Bend your right leg, grab it with both hands just below the knee, and pull it gently toward your chest as far as it will go.

3. Hold your leg at its maximum position for a count of five, making sure your other leg is straight and on the floor.

4. Slowly release and repeat with your left leg. (See Figure 11-10.)

Figure 11-10:
Knee to
chest
stretch. This
stretch is
great for
your lower
back,
buttock
muscles,
and hip joint.

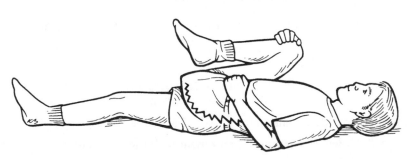

The spinal twist

Exercises that twist the spine are good for maintaining the flexibility of the spine and the oblique muscles — muscles that run diagonally along your side and allow you to reach for something in back of you without completely turning around.

1. Lie on your back on your exercise mat, legs extended and arms at your sides.

2. Bend your right knee and bring it toward your chest, grabbing hold of it with both hands behind the thigh.

3. Extend your right arm straight out to the side, keeping it flat on the floor and making a 90 degree angle to your body.

4. Using your left hand, pull your right knee across your body, as if to touch it to the floor beside your left hip. Your right foot should stay in contact with your left knee and your right shoulder should stay flat on the floor. Your left leg should stay straight.

5. Turn your head to the right, as if looking at the right wall.

6. Hold this pose for a count of 10, then slowly return to your original position.

7. Repeat, bending your left knee this time. One time on each side is sufficient.

The child's pose

This posture stretches your entire back, your buttock muscles and your upper arms, while putting you into a dreamy state of relaxation.

1. Sit on your mat with your legs tucked under you, heels directly under the buttocks. Your knees should be about 12 inches apart.

2. Roll your upper body head first toward the floor, until you can place your forehead on the floor in front of your knees. Place your palms on the floor on either side of your head.

3. Slowly extend your arms in front of you as far as possible. Your buttocks should stay in contact with your heels, and your feet should stay on the floor.

4. Hold this position for a count of 10, then slowly return to the sitting position.

5. Repeat 5 times.

Doing Chair Exercises to Save Your Joints

If you like the idea of exercising without putting a load on your joints, you might consider doing "chair exercises," which are performed while sitting in a straight-back chair. Here are some simple chair exercises that can be used for warm-ups (or, if performed more vigorously, as aerobic exercises):

Chair marching

1. Sit up tall in your chair with feet planted on the ground and pointing straight ahead.

2. "March" your feet in place, beginning slowly then gradually picking up the pace. Be sure to lift your thighs as far off the chair seat as possible.

This is a good one to do with music — try a Souza march! Be careful not to slam your feet on the ground in your enthusiasm, though.

Chair running

This is similar to chair marching but at a much faster pace. It's fair to "run" on your toes (it's too fast a pace to put your whole foot down), and you won't be able to lift your thigh off the chair as high as you do in chair marching. But a couple of minutes of chair running are guaranteed to make you "glow" and start shedding your sweaters.

Chair dancing

You can do the Hora, the Heel-Toe Polka, or Shuffle-Off-To-Buffalo all while sitting in a chair. Not only will it warm you up, it's fun!

The hora

1. Starting with your right foot, step to the side.

2. Cross behind your right foot with your left.

3. Step to the side with your right.

4. Do a small kick with your left foot.

5. Then kick with your right foot.

6. Reverse it: step side with your left, back with your right, side with your left, kick right, kick left.

As with all dancing, the right music can make you forget that you're exercising and feel like you're just kicking up your heels. Music for the Hora can be found in the Jewish folk music section at your local record store.

Heel-toe polka

1. Start with your right foot. Touch your right heel to the floor, then touch your right toe to the floor.

2. Step to your right side with your right foot, then bring your left to meet it.

3. Step to the right again with your right foot.

4. Reverse: Left heel touches, then left toe, step side with left, bring right to meet it, step left.

The count should go: heel, toe, step-together-step, or 1, 2, 1-2-3.

Shuffle-off-to-Buffalo

1. Begin with both feet all the way to the left of your chair. Lift your right foot slightly off the floor and "hop" on your left foot.

2. Step to the side with your right foot.

3. Cross your left behind the right.

4. Step right again, cross left behind.

5. Step right again, cross left behind

6. Step right.

7. Reverse, starting with your left foot.

The sequence goes hop-step, cross, step, cross, step, cross, step, with a count of "and one and two and three and four."

Chair fencing

1. Sitting up straight, extend your right leg forward as far as you can while keeping your foot flat on the floor, toes pointing straight ahead.

2. Extend your right arm forward, in a thrusting position, with left arm against your side, elbow bent and fist curled against the front of your shoulder.

3. Reverse, extending your left leg and left arm. Continue to change positions, as if you were "fencing."

Many more dance steps can be performed from a chair; it only takes a little imagination. Try out some of your favorites; you'll be surprised how enjoyable this kind of exercise can be.

Maximizing the Healing Effects of Exercise

Performing the proper exercises on a regular basis is a vital part of almost any arthritis treatment program. But to gain maximum benefits, you also need to be aware of proper exercise techniques, and always make sure that you're completely warmed up before exercising. A warm bath or shower can help, but you should also do some light cardio or strengthening exercises until you break a sweat. If you have painful, inflamed joints, you may find that icing them before your warm-up helps keep pain at a minimum.

As for exercising when you're in the midst of an arthritis flare, try a warm shower or bath, and then some gentle stretching to get a little circulation going. Take it easy, though. If stretching causes too much pain, stop. You can always try again later.

Warming up your muscles, through light exercise or a warm shower, is just one idea for making the most of your exercise sessions. Here are some other helpful tips:

- ✔ Start slowly with a program that you can do fairly easily.
- ✔ Stop exercising if you feel dizzy, nauseous, faint, or tightness in your chest, and call your doctor.
- ✔ Pick a cardio-endurance activity that you can do continuously for 10 minutes, if possible. (If not, try 5 minutes or even 1 minute, and gradually increase your time.)
- ✔ Make your cardiovascular-endurance exercises vigorous enough so that you sweat, your heart beats faster, and you breath comes more rapidly. Do your cardiovascular endurance exercises three days a week (every other day, with one day off per week) for at least 10 minutes, but not more than 30 minutes.
- ✔ Exercise at a slower pace to cool down after doing cardio-endurance exercises. For example, you can walk slowly until your heart rate returns to normal.
- ✔ Do your strength training exercises three days a week, on the days you don't do cardiovascular endurance exercises. Leave one day a week free for rest.

> ✔ Do some flexibility exercises (stretching) before your strengthening routine, and then again afterwards. This will help decrease the likelihood of injury to the muscles.
>
> ✔ Ask your physical therapist to supervise your stretching sessions, at least in the beginning. Incorrect stretching can cause more harm than good. Stretching sessions should last from 10 to 20 minutes, with each stretch held at least 5 seconds. As you become more flexible, you can gradually increase the holding time to 10, 20, or even 30 seconds. Stretch every day, if possible.
>
> ✔ Always stretch slowly and carefully — don't bounce. Move your body to its maximum position, hold it in place for at least 30 seconds, then ease into your stretch just a little more before releasing.
>
> ✔ Don't hold your breath while stretching — breathe slowly and deeply and try to relax into the stretch.

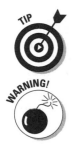

One of the most important things you can do to help make exercise a permanent part of your life is to keep a positive attitude toward yourself, your body, and your program. Remember, the more you exercise, the easier it gets.

Although we've said that exercise may help ease your current joint pain and lessen tomorrow's pain, we don't suggest that you go for a jog when your arthritic knees act up or that you do push-ups when your wrist aches. If an exercise or activity hurts, or causes your joints to become inflamed, *stop immediately*. Pain is a message from your body telling you that tissue is being damaged. Respect the pain; try a different kind of exercise or call it a day and try again tomorrow.

Designing Your Workout Program

You'll become more knowledgeable as you read this chapter, but what you learn by reading this book is not a substitute for professional advice. Doing the wrong exercises, or even the right exercises in the wrong way, can make your condition worse. That's why it's important to enlist professionals to help you design your exercise program so that you do the right exercises in the right way.

Your doctor can advise you as to which kinds of exercise are helpful for your condition, how much is too much, and when to stop. A physical therapist can also be extremely helpful by suggesting appropriate exercises, teaching you correct techniques and positioning, and urging you on when it's time to increase the length and/or intensity of your workout. (An *exercise physiologist* can do much of what a physical therapist does, but make sure that he or she has experience working with arthritis.) And an occupational therapist can teach you how to use your joints in the least stressful ways.

The basic game plan

With the help of your health care professionals, you can begin to devise an exercise plan. The ideal exercise session contains all of the following elements:

- ✔ Warm-up
- ✔ At least 20 minutes of cardiovascular endurance exercises or on alternate days strength-training exercises
- ✔ Flexibility exercises
- ✔ Cool-down

The warm-up

Every exercise session should begin with a thorough warm-up to get the blood circulating and literally increase the temperature of the muscle. This makes muscles more pliable and less likely to be injured. Think of your body as a finely-tuned car. You wouldn't dream of starting up your car, throwing it into gear, and taking off like a shot. Show your body the same consideration as you would your car.

A good warm-up lasts at least ten minutes and should make you break a sweat. If your joints can handle it, calisthenics (jumping jacks, jogging in place, and so on) make ideal warm-up exercises. If not, try doing the slow version of the activity you plan to do next; for example, slow walking or relaxed cycling before beginning a brisk walk or bike trip.

Do not begin your warm-up with big stretches (for example, the hamstring stretch). Stretching a cold muscle invites injury. Save your flexibility exercises until after the bulk of your exercise session has been completed. (A small amount of gentle stretching is okay during the warm-up, but be careful.)

The "Big Three" arthritis exercises

Most people with arthritis tend to gravitate toward three kinds of cardio-endurance exercises — walking, cycling, and water exercises — because they are easy on the joints. You might want to start with these, and then begin to investigate other activities as you get stronger and more adventurous.

Walking

Unless you have severe trouble with your feet, ankles, knees or hips, walking can be an ideal exercise. It's easy, inexpensive (all you really need is a good pair of supportive shoes and some absorbent socks) and can be done just about anywhere. It also provides the weight-bearing exercise you need to keep your bones in shape without the heavy impact on your joints delivered by running or jogging.

In order to get cardio benefits, though, you'll need to work your way up to *brisk* walking. Strolling is certainly pleasant and beneficial, but you'll have to pick up the pace if you want walking to qualify as a true cardiovascular endurance exercise. That means walking fast enough to make you somewhat winded (but not gasping for breath!).

Cycling

Whether you do it by flying through the park on an autumn day or by pumping away in the comfort of your very own bedroom, cycling can be a great way to get your heart racing without putting much strain on your joints. Start on flat ground. Then after several sessions and if your joints permit it, you can raise the level of incline on your stationary bike or find a road that slopes upward slightly as you ride your outdoor bike. Take it easy, though. Strenuous uphill cycling is not recommended for those with osteoarthritis of the knees or hips.

As with walking, you'll need to pick up the pace. Coasting along is certainly pleasant but doesn't count for much if you're trying to give your heart and lungs a workout. If you're riding outdoors, look for a place free of traffic lights, pedestrians and other impediments, since it's hard to get your heart rate up and keep it there if you're forced to stop every two minutes.

Water exercises

Exercising in the water is just what the doctor ordered for most arthritis sufferers: It offers overall physical conditioning and great cardio-endurance with little or no pressure on the joints. With water to buoy you, you can say good-bye to gravity's woes and get your heart pumping without feeling that nagging pain in your knees or hips.

One of the best kinds of exercise that you can do to increase your head-to-toe fitness is swimming. When you swim, more than two-thirds of the muscles in your body go into action, giving you a good total workout in a short time. It's an efficient and enjoyable way to increase your overall strength, endurance, and flexibility – even your posture!

For those who like the water but aren't keen on swimming, water aerobics can be a good choice. Offered by many local YMCAs in conjunction with the Arthritis Foundation, these classes are held in warm-water pools. Those with arthritis or other joint problems are led by a qualified instructor through a series of gentle range-of-motion, cardio-endurance, and flexibility exercises. Many people find that not only is their pain reduced during the time they are in the water, but also both their mobility and relief from pain are increased for hours (or even days) after a workout.

How often and how long?

According to the American College of Sports Medicine, you should do at least 20 minutes worth of continuous cardiovascular endurance exercises at least three times a week. If you haven't exercised in a while, though, or if you're experiencing a lot of joint pain, this might not be possible. The best idea is to start wherever you are right now. If you can only do five minutes worth of aerobic exercises, then so be it. Perhaps by next week you can increase it to six minutes. The point is to get moving and gradually improve.

If you find that you're doing great at your present level and aren't experiencing any physical problems, you can increase the length of your cardio workout and/or the number of sessions you do per week. The maximum is three 30-minute sessions per week. Any more than this isn't going to make much difference in your fitness level, but it will increase your risk of injury.

How do I know if I'm working hard enough?

First of all, as long as you're doing some form of exercise, you should be congratulated! A whopping 50 percent of American adults, many of whom have no excuses, get no exercise at all. If you're at least making an effort, especially on a daily basis, you're definitely on your way to better fitness and better health.

But to get the most out of your cardiovascular endurance exercises without running the risk of exhaustion, you'll need to remember two things while exercising:

- ✔ Your breath should be coming faster and harder, but not to the point where you're panting.
- ✔ Your heart should be beating faster, but not pounding in your ears!

So how do you figure out if you're doing enough, but not too much? Try using the Target Heart Rate system.

1. First, subtract your age from 220. (Example: 220 − 60 = 160)
2. Then, multiply the answer by .9 *and* by .6 (example: 160 x .9 = 144; 160 x .6 = 99).

Your two answers indicate the upper and lower ends of your target heart rate zone. That means that for maximum cardio-endurance benefits, your heart rate should fall somewhere between these two numbers while you're exercising — in this case somewhere between 144 and 99 beats per minute.

To figure your current heart rate, all you need is a watch or clock with a second hand and your own fingers:

- ✔ Place your index and second fingers across the inside of your opposite wrist. There's a little "well" on the thumb-side of the tendon that runs up the middle of your wrist. Your two fingers should easily slide over that tendon and into this "well," where it should be easy to feel your pulse.
- ✔ With an eye on the second-hand of your watch or clock, count the number of pulse beats you feel in 15 seconds.

- ✔ Then multiply by four and you'll have the number of times your heart beats in a minute.

- ✔ If you do this either during or immediately after your cardio-endurance session, you should be able to figure out whether you're in "the zone" or not.

Here's an easy way to find out if you're working hard enough (or too hard) while exercising. You should be breathing too heavily to be able to sing, but not so heavily that you can't talk. If you can sing while you're exercising, you might want to step up the intensity a bit. But if you find you can't catch your breath enough to talk during exercise, you're probably overdoing it.

Take it easy!

Whenever you start a new exercise program, add a new activity, or increase the frequency or duration of your workout, the number one rule is this: Start slowly. Many would-be exercise enthusiasts are sidelined by doing too much too soon, winding up either injured or just plain burned out! Your exercise sessions should emphasize enjoyment. They should require some effort but should never be grueling. If you're more than just a little bit sore a day or two after the workout, you've done too much.

Finding a Good Class

After you've done some initial training with a physical therapist or exercise physiologist, you may feel ready to join a class. There are several advantages to working out in groups — it's a lot less expensive than private instruction, classes usually have more space, and a greater variety of equipment and the friendships formed between classmates can make exercise more fun. But where can you find a class suited to the special needs of those with arthritis? The best bet is to contact your local chapter of Arthritis Foundation and ask about their YMCA Aquatics Program.

The YMCA and the Arthritis Foundation jointly offer a warm-water exercise program at YMCAs and YWCAs nation-wide. The pool is typically kept at about 83 degrees, and often soft music is played in the background. A specially-trained instructor takes the class through a variety of stretching, strengthening and aerobic exercises, and the buoyancy of the water allows participants to increase overall fitness without putting excessive strain on their joints

The Arthritis Foundation also offers exercise videotapes for those with moderate to severe arthritis. The People with Arthritis Can Exercise (PACE) videos take viewers through both range-of-motion and strengthening exercises. Contact your local Arthritis Foundation chapter for more information.

Chapter 12

The Right Stride and Other Ways to Protect Your Joints

In This Chapter

▶ Using your joints in more efficient and less damaging ways

▶ Saving your joints with correct posture

▶ Walking correctly

▶ Sitting in the least stressful, most healthful position

▶ Using ergonomics to reduce fatigue, stress, and injury

*T*he little things you do every day — such as sitting, standing, and walking — and the way you do them can be major factors in determining how healthy or hurtful your joints are today and how well they fare tomorrow.

You may think that sitting in a chair or walking down the street is a natural behavior that you instinctively know how to do correctly. After all, you've been doing these things all of your life. But believe it or not, almost everybody misuses their joints by doing some of these things incorrectly. And, over time, repeated abuse of your joints can cause permanent tissue damage and a lot of unnecessary pain. Luckily, by learning certain joint-saving techniques, you can take undue pressure off your joints today, thereby helping to prevent tomorrow's problems. In this chapter, we tell you how you can take a load off your joints while doing everyday things that you probably don't realize can be harmful.

Excellent Ergonomics

With so many of us permanently wed to the computer, the incidence of neck, back, wrist, and hand problems has risen phenomenally, giving birth to a whole new field of study — *ergonomics*. Ergonomics involves the design of equipment that "fits" the body and allows it to function in its least-stressful positions. As a result, bodily stress, strain, fatigue, and repetitive motion injuries can be reduced.

When sitting at the computer, think 90 degree angles. Your head and torso should be erect, as if a piece of string attached to the top of your head was pulling you toward the ceiling. Your chin, arms, thighs, and feet should make 90 degree angles to your body as you type. See Figure 12-1 for an example.

Remember that angling your neck and head downward to read is stressful to your neck. A book stand or a document holder that attaches to the side of your computer can help you maintain the proper position of your head and neck. When you are sitting at your desk working at your computer, your body should be aligned in the following manner:

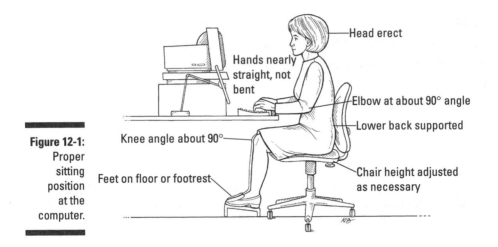

Figure 12-1:
Proper
sitting
position
at the
computer.

Take a look at your workstations (both at work and and home) and see if they meet the following requirements. If not, start making the ergonomically correct changes today!

- ✔ The top of your computer screen should be just below eye level.

- ✔ Your eyes should be 18 to 28 inches away from the screen.

- ✔ Your chin should be at a 90 degree angle to your neck when you look at the screen.

- ✔ Shoulders should be relaxed but not hunched over as you type. Forearms should be at a 90 degree angle to your body and your wrists and hands should be flat (not bent, flexed, or curled) on the keyboard.

> ✔ The chair should have adjustable arm rests that support both your fore-arms and elbows at a 90 degree angle. This eliminates neck strain and postions the wrists properly.
>
> ✔ Lower back should be supported by the chair's built-in lumbar support, a rolled-up towel, or a cylinder-shaped pillow.
>
> ✔ Knees should be bent, creating a 90 degree angle between your upper and lower legs.
>
> ✔ Feet should be flat on the floor.

Save your own neck! Don't hold the phone receiver with your shoulder as you talk. Either hold it with your hand or get a headset.

Even if your workstation is ergonomically perfect, don't sit in one position for too long. Every 15 minutes or so, get up, stretch, and move around a little to get your circulation going and relieve muscular stress and strain. Do some head rolls, shoulder rolls, and neck stretches. Gently stretch your fingers toward the back of your wrist. Shake your arms and hands and let them dangle loose at your side. Your body will thank you for it!

Biomechanics

It's difficult for most people to analyze their own postures or the ways they move, which means it's equally hard for them to figure out just how they may be overstressing their joints. That's why you may want to be evaluated by a practitioner who specializes in biomechanics.

Do your biomechanics need a tune-up?

Biomechanics is the study of how your body handles the impact of its own weight against gravity. When your body is in a "biomechanically correct" position, the force of the impact created by movement is spread out over a large area. During correct walking, for example, when your heel strikes the ground, the impact travels up your entire leg and is absorbed along the way by your foot, ankle, knee, and hip, and all their supporting tissues. But during incorrect walking, the brunt of the impact may be taken by the ankle and knee alone. By distributing the load as widely as possible and positioning the joints for maximum impact absorption, joint stress and damage can be cut.

Learning correct biomechanical (joint-saving) techniques is something *everybody* should do to protect their joints. And for those who already have joint problems, observing correct biomechanics is absolutely essential.

Besides physical therapists and physicians trained in sports medicine or osteopathy, you may want to consider a practitioner trained in one of the following areas to help you with overall body alignment:

- ✔ **The Alexander Technique:** Developed by F. Mathias Alexander, an actor who couldn't shake a lengthy case of laryngitis, the basis of this technique is that faulty posture and poor movement habits contribute to problems in both the physical and emotional realms. (Alexander found that his laryngitis was the result of tension and moving improperly.) Students are taught to stand, walk, and sit in ways that are less stressful to the body through the use of movement, touch, and awareness.

- ✔ **The Feldenkrais Method:** Moshe Feldenkrais, a physicist, martial arts expert, and engineer, devised this method to heal a sports-related knee injury without resorting to surgery. By changing unhealthy movement habits, learning to breathe deeply, and improving the self-image, patients learn how to ease their pain. Classes are held in which patients are taken through exercises that increase flexibility, range of motion, and body awareness.

- ✔ **Trager Approach:** Milton Trager, M.D., believed that stress and pain originate in the mind and that bodywork can change the mental and physical habits that lead to them. Although the Trager Approach is more like massage (you lie on a table and the practitioner manipulates your body), the gentle moving of your body (rocking, stretching, and so on) can help you relax and increase your body-mind awareness.

Although there are no bonafide studies proving that any of these methods work for arthritis, many physical therapists extol their benefits for rheumatoid arthritis, osteoarthritis, and fibromyalgia. In the end, you'll have to decide for yourself whether one of these methods is worthwhile. (Remember that it may take several sessions and a significant investment of time and money before you can come to a decision.) But if one of these methods does make you feel better, great! Just make sure you find a certified therapist (see Appendix B: Resources), listen to your body, and don't do anything that causes you pain.

Standing Tall: Body Alignment

You can start improving your posture right now, just by becoming aware of its general principles. Correct posture is a group effort involving many parts of the body.

You should stand with your feet slightly apart and toes pointing forward or just a little turned out. "Turn out" occurs when the toes point away from the center of the body. If you think of your feet as the hands of a clock, pointing at 12 when they're straight forward, a slight turnout would put your left foot at 11 o'clock and your right foot at 1 o'clock.

You should distribute your weight evenly across your heel, along the inner edge of the outside of your foot, up to the ball of your foot. (Don't walk on the outside "rim" of your foot, but don't transfer your weight in toward your arch, either.) The weight should also be borne by your big toe, second and third toes, and on the ball of the foot directly under the big toe. Figure 12-2 shows an example of the proper distribution of weight on your foot.

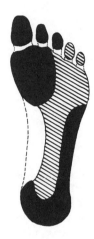

Figure 12-2:
Proper
distribution
of weight on
the sole of
the foot.

Many people carry their weight primarily on the inner edge of their feet, in a line that runs directly from the big toe down to the arch side of the heels. This causes their arches to collapse and their ankles to roll inward or *pronate*. Because the feet and ankles make up the base of the body, pronation throws the alignment out of whack all the way up. (Can you imagine the result if the Eiffel Tower had "pronated ankles"?) Pronation is a major cause of poor posture and, if you pronate, simply trying to stand up straighter won't solve your posture problem. You need to correct the pronation first. (You may need to see a physical therapist to help you accomplish this.)

If you're a pronator, try rolling your weight more toward the outer edge of your feet, but not so far that your big toe is no longer bearing weight. See Figure 12-3 for the correct and incorrect position of your ankles.

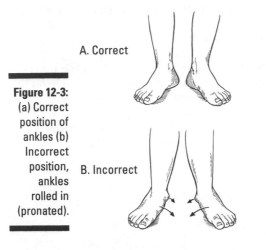

A. Correct

B. Incorrect

Figure 12-3:
(a) Correct position of ankles (b) Incorrect position, ankles rolled in (pronated).

Bent knees

Another cause of misalignment is *locked knees,* in which the front of the knee is completely straight (with no give to it at all) and the back of the knee is swayed back or hyperextended. Many people adopt the locked knees position because it requires less muscular effort to stand this way. Your leg and rear–end muscles aren't really holding you up; your leg bones are just locked into an unbending position. It's as if your upper body is perched on two stilts. The locked knee position is tough on knee joints because it forces them into misalignment, but it's even worse for the lower back, which automatically sways in response.

The locked knees habit is a hard one to break, because most people are completely unaware that they're doing it. If you have this habit, remind yourself to keep your knees slightly bent whenever you're standing, especially for long periods of time. This means when you're standing in line at the grocery store or the bank, and also when you're ironing, doing dishes, waiting for a street light to change, or standing over your child while he or she does homework. It will take a little more effort to stand this way, but you'll build up your "good posture muscles" while you work on healthier joint alignment.

If you're standing in line at the movies, ease the pressure on your knees by shifting your weight subtly back and forth from foot to foot. Don't put all your weight on one foot; just transfer the bulk of the burden. If you find yourself standing for a long time (for instance, while ironing), you may try putting one foot up on a stool, which helps flatten the back and keeps you from slouching.

Lower back

Your pelvic bones should face straight forward like headlights on the front of a car. If yours point slightly downward, you may have a *sway back* — a lower back with an excessive curve. Swaying your back is often the result of locked knees and loose stomach muscles. A major cause of back pain, swaying puts extra pressure on the ligaments, muscles, and joints in your spine.

If you're wondering whether or not you have a sway back, try this test:

1. Stand with your back to a wall, assuming your typical relaxed posture.

2. Slide your hand behind your lower back into the space between your back and the wall.

3. Your hand should almost be able to touch both your back and the wall at the same time.

If there is extra room between your hand and your back, you're probably swaying your back. Try contracting your buttock muscles and tucking them under in order to flatten your lower back. Contracting your stomach muscles helps, too.

Believe it or not, one of the best ways to protect your lower back is to keep your stomach muscles firm and toned. If these muscles are weak, your center of gravity is thrown off, your posture distorted, your back muscles and ligaments strained, and the discs in your lower back unduly stressed. Rather than just "letting it all hang out" when sitting or standing, contract your stomach muscles and tuck your rear-end under. Your posture will improve automatically, the pressure on your lower back will ease, and you'll be giving these muscles a mini workout.

Relaxed shoulders

Your shoulders should line up with your ears — not hunched forward but not pinned back behind you, either. Rounding the shoulders is a common bad habit that lengthens upper back muscles and exaggerates the upper back curve while causing the chest cavity to "cave in." Not only is this hard on the back and neck, it's also a very low-energy position. Your lungs can't fill to capacity when your chest is sunken. Pull your shoulders back to a *midline position* (too far back will throw off your alignment), and press down the area between the neck and the shoulders, lengthening the neck. Raised shoulders are full of tension that will eventually express themselves as neck or back pain.

Holding your head high

Your head weighs anywhere from 10 to 12 pounds, so it's no wonder that your neck may sometimes bow under the strain of holding it up. Your neck should have a gentle forward curve to it that's similar to the shape of a banana. Many people jut their heads forward, though, distorting the natural shape of the neck and putting excessive pressure on certain vertebrae.

The "forward head" is the natural result of the round-shoulders, caved-in-chest position that so many of us assume. To correct this, first pull your shoulders back until they line up with your ears, and open up your chest. Then gently pull your chin in toward your neck — not to the point of making a double chin, but a little more than what feels natural to you. Your eyes should be straight ahead and your chin parallel to the floor as you do this.

Now, put it all together! From stem-to-stern, here are the elements of good posture, the most efficient and least stressful ways to position your body:

- ✔ Head erect, with chin slightly pulled in
- ✔ Neck long
- ✔ Shoulders relaxed and slightly pulled back; they should line up with your ears
- ✔ Buttock muscles slightly tightened to counteract "sway back"
- ✔ Stomach muscles contracted
- ✔ Knees slightly bent
- ✔ Ankles directly over the feet (not pronated)
- ✔ Feet apart, weight evenly distributed across the heels, the first three toes, and the ball of the foot directly under the big toe

Now that you know how to stand correctly, you can do a lot to alleviate uneven wear-and-tear on your joints. But we don't just stand around all day — we move, too! And just as there are joint-saving ways to stand, there are also joint-saving ways to move.

The Right Stride

Our Aunt Bessie used to say, "My mother never taught me to walk correctly, and that's why I have bad ankles today." We all pooh-poohed this idea (although not to her face). How ridiculous! Walking is just putting one foot in front of another. What was Bessie's mother supposed to do, other than get her on her feet and let her go?

Today we know that dear old Aunt Bessie was right — there is a correct way to walk, just as there are loads of incorrect ways. And no matter how natural it may feel to you, if you're walking incorrectly, you're throwing off your body's alignment. The end result is uneven wear-and-tear on your joints, pain, and (sometimes) permanent joint damage. Think of a car that's out of alignment: Eventually some areas of the tires wear smooth, while others still have plenty of traction. If this goes on long enough, the tires become worthless, and you have to buy a whole new set. The same is true of your joints — although buying a whole new set is not usually an option! See Figure 12-4 for the correct position of the feet when walking.

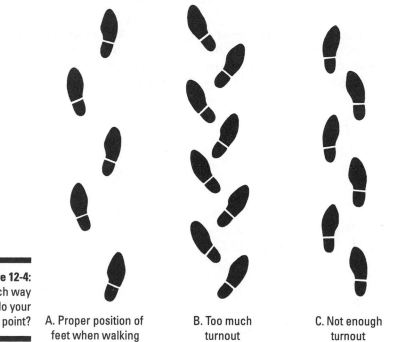

Figure 12-4:
Which way
do your
toes point?

A. Proper position of
feet when walking

B. Too much
turnout

C. Not enough
turnout

Correct walking is based on the principles of good posture with just a few additions:

✔ Turn your feet out slightly, just 15 or 20 degrees (see Figure 12-4). Feet that are turned out more than about 20 degrees (think ballet dancer), pointed straight ahead, or turned slightly inward (think pigeon-toed) will throw off your body alignment.

✔ Make sure your heel is centered as it strikes the ground. (Remember: Avoid "rocking in" on your ankles.)

✔ Feet should be about 8 inches to 10 inches apart as you walk. (Don't cross one foot over the other as you step.)

✔ Keep your knees in an ever-so-slightly flexed position at all times (no "locking back").

✔ Swing your arms naturally as you walk, moving them in a straight line forward and back, not around your body. Palms should face inward toward your thighs.

✔ Keep your head erect, with eyes and chin just slightly lower than horizontal level.

✔ Tilt your body forward, almost as if you are falling toward the front, with your weight on the balls of your feet. This brings your center of gravity forward and helps stamp out the old locked-knees, sway back, stomach-out alignment. See Figure 12-5 for an example.

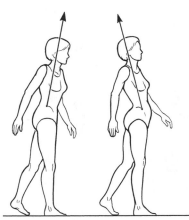

Figure 12-5:
Proper
angle of the
body when
walking.

A. Proper-Upper
body angled forward

B. Improper-Upper
body angled backward

Saving Your Joints While Sleeping

Remember when you were a kid and one of the most fun things in the whole world was to fly through the air and bellyflop on your parents' bed? Well, it goes without saying that's the exact opposite of the way you should lie down today.

The best way to go from upright to lying flat is to

1. Sit on the edge of the bed.

2. Support your body weight by placing your hands flat on the mattress to one side of your body. (You may need to bend one of your arms and lean on your elbow.)

3. Draw your legs up, knees bent, until you can lie on your side.

4. Adjust your arms, legs, and pillows until you are in a comfortable position.

Although most people arise by sitting straight up in bed and then throwing their legs over the side, it's much easier on your joints to

1. Scoot over to the edge of the bed while lying on your side, facing the edge of the mattress.

2. Place your hands flat on the mattress and push yourself up while you simultaneously swing your legs down to the floor. The weight of your legs will counterbalance the weight of your upper body and help pull you to a sitting position.

If you're lying on the floor during an exercise session and you want to sit up, don't just throw your body up in a sit-up position. Roll to your side and push off with your hands. You'll help save your back and your neck in the long run.

Heavy (Or Light!) Lifting

By now, everybody should know that you don't just bend over to pick up a weighty load. This position puts great stress and strain on your back muscles, especially those in the lower back. But if you think about how most people pick up small children, you'll realize that improper lifting goes on all the time.

Lifting any size load (even baby-sized ones) should always be done this way:

1. Make sure the load is as close to your body as possible before lifting it. The further away it is, the greater strain it places on your lower back.

2. Keeping your back straight and your neck in line with your spine, bend your knees until you can get your hands under the load.

3. Use two hands for lifting, instead of one. After you have a good grasp, rise by straightening your legs, keeping your back straight at all times.

Setting a load down should be done in the same way; just reverse the process. And, whenever possible, slide the load along the floor instead of lifting it.

If you feel pain while lifting, you're overdoing it. Stop immediately and find another way to get the job done.

The Seven Keys to Joint Protection

According to the Arthritis Foundation, there are seven ways to protect your joints from injury and/or excessive stress. These seven keys can help you unload a great deal of joint stress and strain, while helping to prevent futher bone and/or tissue damage:

✔ Respect pain.

✔ Avoid improper postures or positions.

✔ Avoid staying in one position for a long time.

✔ Use the strongest and largest joints and muscles for the job.

✔ Avoid sustained joint activities.

✔ Maintain muscle strength and joint range of motion.

✔ Use assistive devices or splints, if necessary.

Chapter 13

Controlling Your Stress, Aggression, and Depression

● ●

In This Chapter

▶ How the brain interprets pain messages

▶ Why the "fight or flight" response may make you hurt

▶ Reducing stress to reduce pain

▶ Slowing down the "Type A" way of life

▶ Fighting depression as a means of fighting pain

▶ Finding an arthritis support group

● ●

*W*e used to believe that pain was simply a matter of a hurting impulse traveling from the "ouch point" up the nerves and to the brain. For example, say the bones in your right knee were rubbing together. The nerves would send a pain message up to your brain, and you'd feel a throbbing, grinding, burning sensation in your knee.

But in 1965, two doctors decided that it wasn't quite that simple. They introduced the Gate Theory of Pain, which suggests there are "gates" along the nerve pathways. Like the locks on a canal, these gates can raise or lower to either let pain messages through or block them. And they *don't* automatically have to open wide to every pain message.

Several factors influence this opening and closing of the gates — including your feelings about pain and your experiences with it. Here are some of the things that get those gates swinging one way or the other:

✔ **The way you think about the pain.** Not only what, when, and where, but also your perception of its intensity, duration, and quality.

✔ **The way you feel about the pain.** Emotions that accompany your pain, such as fear, depression, anger, and despair.

✓ **Your tendency to take action in response to the pain.** For example, whether you tend to isolate yourself from others when you're hurt, immediately take pain pills, or take positive self-help measures.

✓ **Your prior experience with pain.** Memories, comparison of this pain to others, your perception of your own coping ability, and so on.

In other words, there's more to pain than the physical problem at the "ouch point." Your thoughts help determine whether the pain messages race through the gates to the brain, move at a more leisurely pace, or crawl slowly along.

The Psychological Effects of Pain: Why We Hurt More Than We Have to

The bad news is that many of us hurt more than we have to because we're quick to think the unhappy thoughts that help open the gates to pain messages. The good news is that positive thoughts and feelings can close those gates — a little or a lot — and make it harder for the pain messages to get through. Of course, pain is pain, and a brick dropped on your toe hurts. No amount of positive thinking can close the gate on that kind of pain message! But good thoughts can act as healing balms for a fair amount of the chronic pain that comes with arthritis.

Switching from one set of thoughts to another will help reduce your pain, but which thoughts are "good" and which are "bad"? The good thoughts are discussed later in the chapter. Now we focus on what you need to clear out of your mind to help reduce pain, namely a trio of notorious "gate openers": stress, Type A behavior, and depression.

Ratcheting up the pain with stress

Flare-ups of rheumatoid arthritis and certain other forms of arthritis can be (and often are) associated with stress. As a matter of fact, any kind of pain, brought about by any ailment, can be worsened by stress. Reducing and managing stress, then, can be very helpful.

In simple terms, stress is your body's respond to *stressors*. Stressors can be anything that frightens, angers, annoys, scares, or challenges you, or forces you to change or respond to change. Cars about to ram into you are stressors, as is a nasty boss giving you a rough time, illness, the loss of a loved one, and a failed relationship. Even good things, like getting married or having a baby, can be stressors because they force you to respond to challenge or change.

But there's a big difference between stressors and stress. Nasty bosses, illness, and failed relationships are stressors, not stress. You *may* get tense, angry or frustrated; you *may* feel helpless and hopeless when these stressors appear — now you're stressed. On the other hand, you may simply ignore the stressors, laugh them off, or find a calm way to deal with them. The facts are the same, but you're not stressed.

Stress can make the "pain gates" swing wide open. If you respond to the stressors by getting stressed, there's a very good chance that whatever already hurts will hurt more.

Increasing pain the "A" way

People often equate the hectic pace of modern life with stress: You wake up early to get the kids ready for school, hurry to work, race through errands during lunch, drive the kids around, run more errands in the evening, and then scramble to throw together something for dinner, with cell phones glued to our ears all the while. It's no wonder so many of us are "stressed out." Or is it? Several studies suggest that feeling harassed and under pressure are not the problem. Instead, it's anger and hostility.

You may have heard about the Type A personality, the often angry, hostile, hard-driving, competition-loving person who seems to relish going into battle. Unfortunately, anger, hostility, and aggression can trigger stress and open the pain gates wide.

Are you a Type A personality? Do you see yourself in any of the following statements:

- Hate to waste any time?
- Feel like you've always got to be accomplishing something?
- Love to compete with others, just for the fun of winning?
- Often think about your life and accomplishments in terms of dollars earned, cases won, opponents defeated?
- Feel somewhat unsatisfied after each success and immediately begin working for the next?
- Anger easily?
- Always feel like you're behind, that you're racing against the clock?
- Leave little time for hobbies and relaxation, taking work with you on vacation?
- Generally dominate conversations, finding it boring to listen to other people talk about themselves or their interests?

> ✔ Making snap decisions that you "know" are right?
>
> ✔ Often feel like other people are in your way?
>
> ✔ Often find yourself locking horns with others?
>
> ✔ Feel threatened when someone questions your achievements?

If you answered yes to more than a few of the questions, you may be a Type A, and this may be increasing your pain.

Depression means pain

Depression, a common companion to lingering and painful arthritis conditions, can also make your pain feel worse. Unfortunately, many people don't realize that they're depressed because the signs of depression are not always obvious. Besides sadness and feeling "low," other possible symptoms of depression include fatigue, irritability, anxiety, withdrawal, weight gain or loss, disturbed sleeping patterns, brooding, excessive or inappropriate crying, not laughing as much as usual, loss of interest in formerly pleasurable activities, feelings of worthlessness or hopelessness, difficulty concentrating, thinking slowly, speaking slowly, and loss of sexual desire or pleasure.

Any these symptoms can and do strike us all from time to time; we all get the blues. But when several of these symptoms strike day after day for a couple weeks or more, it's considered depression.

A fair number of people suffering from chronic arthritis pain become depressed. That's not surprising, given that doctors are unable to cure the disease. This is doubly unfortunate. First, depression itself can be debilitating, sapping our precious physical strength and draining the joy from life. Second, depression can make everything hurt even more. Indeed, in some cases we wonder which is causing more pain: the original arthritis or the resulting depression.

The Healing Power of Positive Thinking

Stress, Type A behavior, and depression can change your perception of pain, pushing the pain gates open and making you hurt more than you have to. That's one of the reason's why doctors have trouble dealing with pain: They can tell how much cartilage has been worn away and can guess how much it *should* hurt, but they can't know whether your attitude toward pain is making the pain greater or lessening the pain.

The good news is that positive thinking can help you close those gates, a little or a lot. Thinking positively doesn't mean you have to love everyone you meet and everything that happens to you. You can be a positive thinker and still get upset now and then, and you can avoid people or situations you don't like. In fact, letting off a little steam once in a while or staying away from annoying people can be a good idea. This section contains a few ideas for relieving pain by reducing stress, lessening Type A behavior and anger, and combating depression.

Reducing pain by reducing stress

Eliminating stress is not a panacea; it won't magically make all your pain disappear. But controlling your stress can help ensure that you don't hurt any more than you absolutely have to — and most of us *do* hurt more than is necessary.

Fortunately, you can help close the pain gates by simply changing the way you think. Reshaping your view of events and taking a more positive approach that calms your reaction to stressors can help you reduce your stress and pain. Remember that you're always going to face stressors, many of which you can't do anything about. But you can always change your attitude toward these stressors.

The next few sections present a few of the many stress-reduction techniques you can use. Which approach is best for you? The one that works. Give them all a try; the ones that help you control your stress and your pain most effectively are the ones you should use.

Stress increases pain by opening the pain gates. To lessen or prevent physical pain, figure out how to reduce and control your stress. Any technique that helps you do this acts like a medicine in your body.

Biofeedback: The thinking approach

Although the body usually runs things as it sees fit, it's possible to override some of its instructions. Biofeedback operates on the premise that "seeing" what's happening inside your body may help you control it. During biofeedback sessions, you're hooked up to sensitive electrical equipment that monitors your blood pressure, heart rate, muscle tension, body temperature, and so on. The machine(s) may beep every time your heart beats, or perhaps a light flashes. A continuous display may show fluctuations in your body temperature or blood pressure, and lights may change colors in response to changes in your skin temperature.

These numbers, displays, lights, and beeps give you something tangible to work with as you learn to control what's happening inside your body. After learning relaxation and visualization techniques, you may be able to alter these bodily functions for the better — and see the results on the monitors. For example, with practice many people can learn to lower their heart rates and otherwise calm themselves, even while in the midst of stress.

Biofeedback is a wonderful teaching tool that gives immediate reinforcement as you practice relaxation techniques. Later, you should be able to apply these techniques in your daily life without the equipment.

You can find a biofeedback practitioner in the yellow pages or by contacting the Association for Applied Psychophysiology and Biofeedback (See Resources.) It's best, however, to get a referral to a biofeedback technician from your physician. Your HMO or insurance plan may have a list of biofeed-back technicians.

Quieting stress with meditation and programmed relaxation

Practiced in many different forms, meditation helps you quiet both your body and your mind. Some forms of meditation are exotic, using chants, incense, and foreign terms, while others are plain and simple. But all forms have one thing in common: a strong, deliberate focus on something outside of the self, such as a mantra (a specific word). You focus strongly on the word (repeating it over and over again in your mind) as a way of keeping your mind still. As thoughts and images drift into your mind, you simply ignore them and concentrate on your mantra. Soon, they'll just drift right out again.

Meditation reduces stress by giving you time away from your thoughts and problems — especially from stressors.

Programmed relaxation, also known as the relaxation response, is another form of meditation. But instead of focusing on a mantra, you tune in to your muscles, feeling them tighten and relax in a programmed manner. Programmed relaxation can help relieve the stress that accompanies chronic pain, reduce your overall pain load, and help you sleep better.

You can learn about meditation and programmed relaxation from many sources, including psychologists and other mental health experts and meditation centers. Some HMOs and hospitals offer courses in meditation, and some large companies offer them for their employees. You can also find a meditation or programmed relaxation practitioner through the yellow pages or by contacting the organizations listed under "Mind/Body Connection" in Appenix B, Resources.

Guided imagery/hypnosis: moving to a stress-free place

Although there is no hard scientific data to prove that guided imagery can dramatically change body chemistry and conditions, many people have benefited from finding out how to put themselves in a better place by imagining happy scenarios. For example, you may imagine yourself relaxing on a beautiful tropical beach when you're actually caught in bumper-to-bumper, rush-hour traffic. You manage to remain calm, at ease, and even happy while those around you are ready to scream with frustration.

The same effect can be accomplished with hypnotherapy. Hypnosis will not cure arthritis, but it can help you handle emotional upsets caused by pain and can help relieve the pain to a certain extent. Hypnosis can help you relax in the face of pain and stress, reduce your stress and anxiety, and make you feel as if you're no longer prisoner to your pain.

You'll find hypnotherapists listed in the Yellow Pages, or you can contact the organizations listed under Hypnotherapy in Appendix B: Resources. The best approach, however, is to get a referral from your doctor or psychologist. (Many psychologists practice guide imagery and hypnotherapy.)

Controlling your breathing

Think about your breathing when you're stressed: You probably take short, shallow breaths. But when you breathe in the opposite manner, with long, deep breaths, your body naturally moves toward a relaxation state. Making it a point to breathe slowly and deeply when you feel stressed can help short-circuit the stress cycle. And by focusing on your breath rather than your fear, frustration, anger or pain, you can also help derail negative feelings.

Laughter

Undoubtedly, the most fun stress reliever is laughter. A good, hard laugh is believed to lower the levels of cortisol, one of the stress hormones. It also helps you relax all over. Laughing takes your thoughts away from whatever is going wrong in your life, so you can't stew in your own negativity. In fact, many health experts believe that a good sense of humor is like a vitamin for both body and soul.

Forgetting all about it

Even something as simple as distracting yourself from your problems can be helpful. Instead of focusing on your pain, which will only increase your stress, try going for a walk with a friend, doing an arts and crafts project, volunteering, going to a sing-a-long, taking a fun class, watching an interesting movie or television show, reading an engrossing book, or listening to some great music. Distraction doesn't cure arthritis, but it does help prevent the stress caused by focusing on pain.

Letting go of Type A behavior and anger helps lessen pain

If you're a Type A, the odds are that you can't simply stop acting that way. You can, however, do quite a bit toward reducing your hostility and calming both yourself and your body chemistry. Try integrating the following behaviors into your busy life:

- Slow down!
- Make it a point to find someone or something to admire every day.
- Take time each day to relax — really relax, not just move your work to a nicer environment.
- Make loved ones and friends a top-of-the-list priority.
- Go easy on others.
- Go easy on yourself.
- Have some fun!
- Accept things you can't change.

Lifting your mood to ease your pain

If you have arthritis or any other painful condition, it's wise to guard against depression and to look for ways to feel that you're in control of your situation and your life. Developing a feeling of control when you've been sabotaged from within by arthritis can be difficult.

Some cases of depression fade away over the course of several months. But don't rely on time as a medicine if you suspect that you are depressed. Depression can increase the sensation of pain, weaken the immune system, and sap your ability to cooperate with treatment and rehabilitation.

There is no instant cure for depression. However, there are steps you can take to help lift your mood.

- **Express your feelings.** Don't pretend everything is all right to please your doctor. If you're frustrated or angry because you're stuck with arthritis and its resultant pain, say so. This doesn't mean that you should misbehave, throw temper tantrums, or break things. Look instead for the middle ground between bottling up your feelings and blowing your top.

In other words, express yourself in an assertive, yet moderate and positive way. Tell your doctor what hurts and ask for help. If a certain pill or procedure doesn't help, say so and ask for another approach. Tell your family if your pain is preventing you from performing your normal activities and ask for help and understanding. It can also be very helpful to join a support group and express your feelings there. (See "Joining an Arthritis Support Group" later in this chapter.)

✔ **Don't get caught to in the "Love Me Because I Hurt Syndrome."** Some depressed people start to subconsciously enjoy what they consider the "good" parts of being depressed (for example, you get lots of sympathy, you're excused from certain chores, you're allowed to act out, you may be given extra treats, and so on). Don't get attached to these secondary gains from depression. Remember, depression can breed more depression, so it's vital that you break the cycle as soon as possible.

✔ **Exercise regularly, even when you don't feel like it.** Take brisk walks, ride a bicycle, or otherwise rev up your body and your body chemistry to increase the production of endorphins, the natural "feel good" hormones.

✔ **Try to avoid seeing yourself as a victim of some horrible disease.** Some forms of arthritis are still mysterious to us, but they are physical diseases, not curses or black magic. New breakthroughs are constantly happening; new therapies and drugs are constantly being developed. At the very least, you can manage your disease. And there's always hope that someone will discover a cure in the near future.

✔ **Walk, talk, and act positively!** Even if you don't feel good, approach life with a positive attitude. If possible, don't shuffle. Instead, walk tall and with vigor. Don't mumble; speak clearly and enthusiastically. Don't look down at your feet; look up. Don't avoid other people's gazes; look them straight in the eye. Even if you're only pretending, always walk, talk, and act positively. You may be surprised to find that soon you're not acting any more — you're really feeling better.

Prayer and Spirituality

Several studies have shown that people who belong to religious groups and regularly attend services are less depressed and anxious than those who do not. Studies with hospitalized patients support the notion that religion is an antidepressant. We can't be certain why this is so, but it may be because being religious makes you feel that someone very important (a higher power) is looking out for you; that you belong to something large and wonderful; that you have a role to play in life; that you are loved; and that you belong to a community of people who can help support you. You can also find plenty of opportunities to help others through your church, temple, or mosque; there's nothing like reaching out to others to help you forget about your own pain and feel better about yourself.

Hand-in-hand with religion goes prayer, which itself is often an antidote to stress. The simple act of praying can relieve stress, and the thoughts expressed in many prayers can also have a calming effect. A favorite of many is the Serenity Prayer: "God grant me the serenity to accept the things I cannot change, the courage to change the things I can, and the wisdom to know the difference."

Of course, you needn't be religious to be spiritual. Spirituality is the quest for a connection with a higher power, however you define that. It's also a search for meaning in life, an attempt to understand the world and your place in it. You can express your spirituality through religion, or you can find your own path. Some people approach spirituality through meditation or yoga. For others, it's communing with nature, writing poetry, or doing charitable deeds. The road to spirituality that you take is yours to choose; you may even define a new one all your own. However you approach spirituality, you may find it a helpful balm for your pain.

Dealing with "Helpful" Loved Ones

Writing in the November/December, 1999 issue of *Arthritis Today,* Mary Dunkin describes the types of helpful loved ones who may be driving you crazy with their advice. Beware of the following types:

✔ **The caretaker:** This person hates to see you suffering and tries desperately to get you to try one treatment after another. Your desires take second place to the caretaker's need to see you well again. The caretaker loves you but can drive you crazy.

✔ **The blamer:** This is the person who insists that things would be much better if only you stopped doing certain things or thinking certain thoughts. The blamer may be attempting to relieve him or herself of responsibility of helping you by pretending everything would be all right if only you would shape up.

✔ **The evangelist:** This "helpful" person absolutely, irrevocably, and unshakably *knows* exactly what will cure you — and insists that you try it. Perhaps the evangelist believes he or she was cured by the same thing, is making money off the therapy, knows someone who was cured by this method, or just believes in it.

✔ **The minimizer:** This is the one who suggests a very simple cure for your complex problem. The minimizer promotes a therapy that's obviously way too simple, perhaps because he or she wants to believe that there are always simple answers to every problem.

✔ **The busybody:** This person is a control-freak who thinks he or she can solve everyone's problems, if they'd just listen.

What do you say to the caretaker, blamer, evangelist, minimizer, and/or busy-body (and everyone else who offers unwanted advice)? Gently but firmly tell them that you appreciate their concern, but you're following your doctor's advice. If they're really annoying, you can say, "Thanks for your concern, but I've got my own thoughts about my illness. Please respect my wishes and allow me to handle it my way."

Joining an Arthritis Support Group

Support groups are as individual as the people who join them. Some are more structured, emphasizing education, while others stress emotional support and the sharing of experiences. Some may be designed for those with a particular kind of arthritis, such as osteoarthritis or rheumatoid arthritis, while others are all-inclusive.

There is generally a leader, who may be either a medical professional (for example, a doctor, nurse, psychologist, or social worker) or simply a member of the group. Groups run by their members are often called self-help or peer groups.

If you think you'd like to try a support or self-help group, keep in mind that it may take some detective work and a sizable investment of time before you find the one that's right for you. Visit several groups and go to each one at least twice. The one-time meeting you observe might be an "off" night for an otherwise dynamic and helpful group. (Or a "good" night for an otherwise disorganized and not very helpful group.)

One of the great things about support groups is they remind you that you're not alone! You needn't try to master all the arthritis terms and treatments by yourself, because thousands of experts are waiting to help you. Who are these experts? Other people who have arthritis, like the ones in your group.

What to expect from an arthritis support group

Joining an arthritis or pain support group can be both educational and comforting. Within these groups, you can find the following:

- A chance to talk about your feelings
- A good reason to get out of the house and interact with people
- Encouragement
- Information

- People who can tell you what to expect from a certain test or treatment, because they've already been through it
- People who understand exactly what you're feeling
- Role models, people who are much more "advanced" in their arthritis than you are, but are living happy, productive, and wonderful lives.
- Sympathy

Finding a support or self-help group

To find a support or self-help group (or a pool of groups from which to choose), ask the members of your health care team for referrals. You can also call the Arthritis Foundation at 800-283-7800, or contact any of the other arthritis organizations in Appendix B. If all else fails, you may try looking in the Yellow Pages under *Psychologists' Information & Referral Services.* Someone listed there may know of an arthritis support group in your area.

And for those of you who don't want to leave the comfort of your desk, there are support groups available on the Internet, including www.arthritiswebsite.com, www.Support-Group.com, and www.dejanews.com. If you want more information on support groups online, write to The American Self-Help Clearinghouse, St. Claire's Hospital, Denville, NJ 07834-2995. The Clearinghouse can help you locate a self-help group or start one of your own.

Chapter 14

Day-to-Day Living with Arthritis

. . . .

. . . .

*A*rthritis or not, you have a life to live! Like everybody else, you probably have a lot on your plate — a job, family responsibilities, household and gardening chores, a social life, a romantic life, pets, hobbies, and maybe more. But there are some days when pain and fatigue, the twin demons, may make you wonder if you can even make it into the next room. On these days, it's particularly important that you find the most efficient, least stressful ways of accomplishing whatever you need to do. But don't wait until you're having a rough day before beginning to think about how to simplify your life. Start today by making a list of the things that you typically need to accomplish each day. Then read this chapter to find ways to take on those tasks with greater ease and efficiency. Jot down ideas as you read and start to make a plan.

Studies have shown that people who take an active part in managing their arthritis and find new ways to cope with physical disabilities do better and feel less pain and fatigue. Don't let yourself be sidelined as life's parade marches by! In this chapter, we show you how to wrest control of your life away from arthritis by applying these three watchwords to your daily activities: *organization*, *planning ahead*, and *prioritizing*. You may be surprised at how much you can accomplish and how good you can feel about yourself, even on a bad day.

Visit an Occupational Therapist

The occupational therapist (OT), a vital part of your treatment team, helps you get through your everyday activities despite your arthritis. A licensed health care professional, the OT interviews and examines you to determine how your arthritis affects the things you do on a daily basis, such as getting into and out of bed, dressing, grooming, eating, drinking, cooking, getting around, shopping, doing housework, and working.

After the OT gets a sense of where and when you may be having trouble, he or she can come up with ideas and recommendations. An OT can design splints or supports that conform to affected body parts, recommend and locate a wealth of assistive devices, and come up with plans to help you get through the day with greater ease and efficiency. The OT can also teach you joint-protection techniques that reduce joint strain and help prevent further damage.

Many people are tempted to skip occupational therapy, thinking it's not really necessary. But those who do will cheat themselves of a great opportunity to attack the practical problems posed by arthritis. Even though medical attention and physical therapy are vital parts of the treatment program, they don't help you figure out how you're going to change a light bulb in the ceiling when you can't raise your arm, or how to get yourself a decent meal when you can barely shuffle around the kitchen. That's why occupational therapy exists — to help you discover easier, more efficient ways of getting through the day. But possibly the most important thing that occupational therapy can teach you is how to conserve your energy.

Conserving Your Energy

Let's face it — even if you're the most organized person in the world and you follow absolutely every principle of arthritis management, you only have so much energy. After that runs out, you're like a car that's out of gas — you have to pull over and stop. Don't waste your precious energy; conserve it so you have the "gas" to get through they day's most important tasks.

The Arthritis Foundation suggests the following ideas for conserving your energy:

✔ **Balance activity with rest.** Don't try to do everything at once; work in some breaks between activities. When tackling chores, don't do two difficult ones in a row. Alternate heavy chores with light ones. In the long run, you'll accomplish more tasks and experience less fatigue by pacing yourself.

✓ **Plan ahead.** Find shortcuts, combine activities that can be done simultaneously, figure out what you can skip, and organize the execution of tasks for maximum efficiency.

✓ **Do the most important things first.** If something absolutely *has* to be done, do it first to make sure it doesn't fall by the wayside as your energy wanes.

Getting a Good Night's Sleep

The best fatigue-fighter in the world is a good night's sleep. If you sleep well, you'll find yourself better able to handle pain, less stressed and depressed, and more energetic. Unfortunately, many people develop trouble sleeping as they grow older, especially if they're suffering from pain. To give your body the best possible chance of a good night's sleep, follow these sleeping guidelines:

✓ **Go to bed and get up at the same time every day (even on weekends).** Getting up at 7:00 a.m. Monday through Friday, but at 10:00 a.m. on Saturday and Sunday, throws off your body's internal clock.

✓ **Keep your sleeping area as dark and as quiet as possible.** Block the light with heavy drapes or blackout shades. Get a white noise machine or turn on a fan to cover up noises that may disturb your sleep.

✓ **Make sure your mattress and pillow are comfortable.** A mattress that is either too hard or too soft and a pillow that doesn't support your head and neck comfortably can interfere with your sleep more than you may realize. If you think you need to make a change, there are loads of options. Ask your OT for recommendations.

✓ **Use your bed for sleep and sex only.** Some people use their beds as the Grand Central Station of their lives — they eat, watch TV and videos, pay bills, read, play with the kids, do office work, and perform beauty routines while firmly ensconced between the sheets. Then they wonder why they can't fall asleep there, too. Your bed should be associated with just two activities — sex and sleeping. It should be the place you go to relax, not to get on with the business of living.

✓ **Get some exercise every day, but not in the latter part of the evening.** Exercising after dinner tends to "rev up" your body, making it harder to fall asleep. Finish your heavy exercise by about 6:00 p.m. (Light exercise, like a stroll or some yoga before bedtime, is fine.)

✓ **Relax for about an hour before bedtime.** Yoga, meditation, reading, a warm bath, listening to soft music or a relaxation tape — all of these are good relaxing activities to help you wind down before going to sleep. Don't try to do 101 chores before falling into bed. You may be exhausted, but your mind will be racing and unable to relax.

✔ **Stay away from caffeine in the evening (this includes coffee, tea, soft drinks, and cocoa).** Caffeine is a stimulant and can keep you awake, even if you ingested it hours earlier. A good rule of thumb is to avoid caffeine after 6:00 p.m.

Using Assistive Devices

One of the best ways to conserve your energy and keep from putting undue stress and strain on your joints is to use assistive devices — equipment that can make performing a task easier, safer, and/or more comfortable, especially when your arthritis is acting up. Assistive devices run the gamut from long-handled shoehorns to hydraulic seat lifts that boost you out of a chair, from bathtub benches to computerized wheelchairs. Some of these devices may require professional installation, others are ready to use upon purchase. You can find many assistive devices at medical supply houses and in mail-order catalogues, or your occupational therapist can steer you to reputable sources. The hardest part will probably be deciding which ones are right for you, and your OT also can help you with that task. Here's a partial list of what's currently available:

✔ **Bathing and grooming:** Bath and shower grab bars, toilet safety frames, bathtub benches, foam tubing for handles (for example, toothbrush, hair brush, and so on), raised toilet seats, toothpaste tube squeezers, long-handled bath sponges, and makeup and razor holders are just a few items that can make bathing and grooming easier to accomplish.

✔ **Dressing:** Button hooks, zipper pulls, sock aids, long-handled shoe horns, shoe removers, cuff extenders, stretch shoe laces, and watch winders can help simplify dressing.

✔ **Food preparation & eating:** Large grip utensils (knives, carrot peelers, silverware, and so on), jar openers, can openers, pull-tab can openers, plastic bag openers, non-slip grips for plates and cups, easy-hold cups, and glass holders (with two handles) can aid in meal preparation and eating.

✔ **General household:** Doorknob turners, key turners, car door openers, faucet turners, voice-activated telephones or speaker phones, telephone headsets, voice-activated computer programs (for correspondence), reachers (long-handled devices that grab items), grips for phone receiver, and long-handled sponges and dusters for cleaning can make the handling of household tasks much easier.

✔ **Getting around:** Canes, crutches, stair walkers, walkers, portable stools, scooters, and wheelchairs can help you become more mobile.

For a list of mail order catalogues featuring assistive devices, see Appendix B, Resources.

Home Caregivers

For those who live alone and don't have the luxury of assistance from family and friends, there are several ways to handle personal care, household, gardening, and transportation chores without trying to do it all yourself. Home health care workers can come to your home and help you dress, bathe, do housework, prepare meals, get to the doctor's office, or just about anything else you can imagine. Housekeepers and gardeners can take care of cleaning, laundry, and yard work. But if that kind of help is too pricey, look to the less expensive sources of assistance. Teenagers (either your own or your neighbor's) are often willing to do yard work or other chores for a small fee. A stay-at-home parent in your neighborhood may be willing to make some extra money by preparing meals or taking you to the doctor. Your church or synagogue may have volunteers who are willing to help you out for free. And your doctor, social worker, or other health-care team workers may be able to refer you to various nonprofit organizations that can offer either inexpensive or free services. Just ask!

Coping with Disability in the Workplace

Many of us spend our workdays in an office, sitting down. It sounds easy, but working on a computer, handling correspondence, and doing other paperwork can be difficult if your hands hurt or it's hard to sit comfortably in a chair. Look into these ideas for streamlining paperwork and making desk duties easier:

- Large scissors with well-padded handles can make cutting easier.

- Roller-ball pens glide more easily across the paper than ballpoint or felt-tip pens.

- A rubber grip that fits around the barrel of a pen or pencil makes it easier to hold and less likely to slip.

- Rubber fingers (they look like a thimble made of rubber) can help you turn pages or thumb through a sheaf of papers without fumbling. Or you can twist a rubber band around the end of your finger for the same effect.

- Seam rippers are a nice substitute if you have trouble handling scissors.

- Tape dispensers with some weight and rubberized bottoms make it easier to pull off a piece of tape using just one hand because they won't move.

If you have Internet access and your employer doesn't object to your handling some office tasks with online business transactions, you can cut down on the time you have to stand in long lines (putting strain on your joints) by doing the following:

- Bank by computer or through the mail. Find out if your bank offers these services. (Most do.)
- Buy your stamps online (www.stampsonline.com) or through the mail. (Call your local post office for details.)
- Buy books, vitamins, gifts — even houses and cars on-line. The days of pounding the pavement to do your shopping are gone!

What about Disability Benefits?

If you can no longer do the kind of work you've been accustomed to doing, you may be eligible for disability insurance benefits. To apply, get a claim form from your doctor, hospital, or your local Employment Development Department Office. Your doctor will need to state the exact nature of your medical condition, and affirm that in his opinion you are unable to work at your present job. But getting disability benefits doesn't mean you can't work at all. If you don't relish the idea of sitting at home, there is a special program run by the Social Security Administration that can help you find a job suited to your abilities while you continue to collect your disability benefits. Your local Social Security office can provide you with more details.

If You're Pregnant . . .

Becoming pregnant when you've got arthritis can affect your body in several ways. You may find that your joints are less stable and "looser." The additional weight may increase symptoms of osteoarthritis to the knee. Your back will tend to sway in response to the additional weight of the baby, so back pain, muscle spasms, or a numbness and tingling in your legs can occur. An increase in water weight can increase stiffness in the hips, knees, ankles (the weight bearing joints) and worsen carpal tunnel syndrome.

On the bright side, some forms of arthritis seem to improve during pregnancy. Rheumatoid arthritis, for example, often improves before the beginning of the fifth month, with a decrease in joint swelling. Sometimes lupus and scleroderma improve as well. However, it is quite possible that you'll experience a flare soon after the birth of the baby.

It's advisable that you see both an obstetrician and a rheumatologist during the course of your pregnancy. You should also continue to take your arthritis medicines (if advised to do so by your doctors), exercise to keep your weight under control, your joints flexible and your muscles strong, follow a nutritious eating plan, observe the rules of joint protection, and use stress management techniques to control mood swings and encourage relaxation.

Making Household Chores Easy

Back in the '60s there was a popular household cleaner that claimed it was so fast and versatile it could whip through your house like a "white tornado," cleaning everything in sight in no time at all. Although the tips that follow won't exactly make a "white tornado" out of you, they will cut the time and effort you spend on household chores. Remember to spread your chores out; don't try to get the whole house clean in one day!

If bending over while doing chores is difficult for you, here are some ways to make cleaning easier:

- ✔ Use tools with long handles whenever possible. A long-handled mop can be used to clean the bathtub or shower, a long-handled feather duster can get those cobwebs out of the corner, and floor wax can be laid down evenly with a long-handled paint roller.

- ✔ If it's easier for you to sit while sweeping, cut down the length of your broom handle or use a child's broom. The broom will do a better job of collecting dust and dirt if the bristles are sprayed with water or furniture polish first.

- ✔ For a dirty bathtub, mix together ½ cup of automatic dishwashing detergent and 2 cups of hot water. Plug the tub, add the mixture and swirl it around with a long handled mop. Let it stand for 20 minutes, then rinse thoroughly with cold water from the shower.

- ✔ Stop bending over to plug and unplug your vacuum cleaner! Add a 30-foot extension cord instead.

If you have arthritis in your hands, you want to eliminate chores that involve scrubbing and "elbow grease" or intricate movements. Here are a few things you can do:

- ✔ Cleaning the fireplace is a dirty, unpleasant job, but you can make it easier if you line the fireplace with aluminum foil before you put in the grate and add the wood. Once the ashes have cooled, spritz them with water (to keep ashes from flying), remove the grate, carefully pull the foil toward you and put the whole mess in the trash!

- ✔ Instead of scrubbing a pot that has burned-on food, sprinkle ½ cup baking soda in the pot, add a cup or two of water and simmer for 20 minutes. Allow to stand for 2 hours. The burned part should wipe right off.

- ✔ If clutching a dusting rag hurts your hands, try putting old socks on both hands, spraying with a small amount of furniture polish, then wiping off table tops and counters with ease.

✔ Use the pointed tip of a can opener to open boxes of hot cereal mix with a "press here" type of opening or to get the metal spouts started on boxes of nonfat milk powder.

✔ Instead of the traditional lace-up style of tennis shoes, try the kind with Velcro closures.

✔ If you can find them, get kitchen utensils (carrot peelers, can openers, stirring spoons, and so on) with extra large, rubber-covered handles for easier gripping.

✔ Foam pipe insulation is great for covering the handles of tools to make them easier to grasp. You can find it in the hardware store in several sizes and slip it on the handles of your knives, carrot peelers, screwdrivers, mops or anything else that has a tendency to slip out of your hands.

You can also make your kitchen more functional and personalized for you. This will make your daily tasks easier and help you cope. Here are a few ideas:

✔ Screw a cup-hook underneath one of your cupboards and use it to pry open pull-tab cans. (You need to get the pull-tab started before the hook can grab it. Slide a dinner knife or spoon under the tab and push it up slightly.)

✔ Put Lazy Susans (turntables) on your refrigerator shelves, in your cupboards and in any other storage areas. This eliminates reaching, straining, and shuffling things around as you try to get an item that's in back.

✔ If dialing a phone is difficult, get a phone with an extra-large keypad or use a pencil to push the buttons. Most phones offer an automatic dial feature so you can call frequently dialed numbers with the touch of a button.

✔ Single arm faucets (the kind often found in kitchens that let you control the temperature and the amount of water with just one lever) are easiest to use and don't require two hands. Consider getting your kitchen and bathroom faucets converted to this style. If you want to keep your double arm faucets, try getting wing-type handles that can be operated with your hand, wrist, or forearm.

It's also easy to make other areas of your home easier to manipulate and deal with on a daily basis by doing the following:

✔ If you have trouble closing the door behind you, install two cup hooks — one in the door, near the doorknob, and one in the door frame, just outside the hinge area. (Position the cup hooks so they are level with each other.) Run a string or elastic cord between the cup hooks. You now have a cord that's easy to grab and will pull the door shut behind you.

> ✔ Wrap rubber bands around a doorknob that is difficult to turn. This will give you a better grip.
>
> ✔ Try using a beaded seat cover on your car seats. The beads roll and make it easier for you to get in and out of your car and then to adjust yourself after you settle in.

P.S. What About Your Sex Life

A survey conducted by the National Council on Aging found that nearly half of those over the age of 60 have sex at least once a month, and a majority of older people feel that sex is an important part of life at any age.

Having arthritis doesn't mean you can't have a romantic relationship. Yet you may find that sex takes a back seat when you're trying to manage pain, medication, emotional issues, and physical limitations. You may have become more dependent on your partner, which can change the nature of your relationship. Perhaps physical limitations and/or deformities caused by arthritis have altered your self-image. Medications may put a damper on sexual desire or performance.

You may also be worried that physical lovemaking will be painful: This alone can cause a lack lubrication and/or orgasm in women, and problems getting and maintaining an erection in men. Both partners may be acutely aware of the "pain factor," and even when everything seems to be going along okay, as soon as one partner winces, the other immediately becomes concerned rather than desirous. Lubrication stops, erections disappear, and the thought of sexual relations goes out the window.

Fortunately, satisfying and pleasurable sex is indeed possible for those with arthritis. The most important thing is to focus on the intimacy and closeness that sexual relations can bring, rather than on some pre-ordained standard of performance. Gentle stroking, kissing, caressing, and massage are wonderful ways of expressing sexuality and nurturing at the same time. In most cases, intercourse is also possible, although it may require careful positioning and gentle technique. To help make sex easier and more pleasurable, try the following suggestions:

> ✔ Take a warm bath beforehand to relax your joints and muscles and ease pain. This can also help increase circulation to your fingers and toes, which is particularly important for those with Raynaud's. (Light exercise and stretching may help, too.)
>
> ✔ Take your pain medication so that it kicks in before your session.

✔ Some medications can bring on chemical imbalances that cause yeast infections. If you get one of these infections, ask your doctor to prescribe treatment.

✔ Talk to your partner about what feels good and what doesn't. Explore various methods of achieving mutual satisfaction. Good communication is an important part of any sexual relationship but is vital when there are difficulties. If you have problems that you and your partner can't seem to resolve by yourselves, seek help from a counselor, doctor, or nurse experienced in dealing with the problems of living with arthritis.

Part IV

Is Alternative Medicine for You?

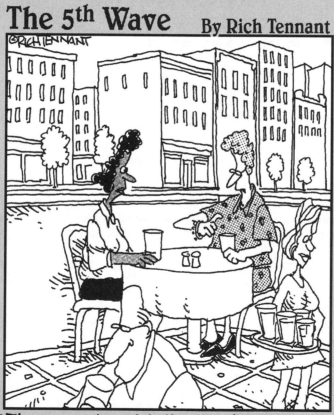

The 5th Wave   By Rich Tennant

"The copper bracelet therapy didn't alleviate my pain, but the diamond and sapphire bracelet therapy seems to be working."

In this part . . .

If the treatment of arthritis were as straightforward and effective as, say, getting rid of a mild headache (that is, take two aspirin and forget it), alternative therapies might not be so popular. Because medical doctors don't offer a real "cure" for arthritis, up to 60 percent of those who suffer from this disease are turning to alternative medicine. Some feel that traditional methods just aren't working, others want help with pain relief and additional symptoms, while still others believe that they really can find a cure if they just look hard enough.

In this part, we discuss the most popular alternative therapies for arthritis, from herbs and homeopathy to "hands on" healing methods, from traditional Chinese medicine to Ayurvedic healing, and everything in between.

Chapter 15

Maneuvering Through the Maze of Miracle Cures

• •

• •

*A*lternative medicine is going mainstream — well, sort of, and only a tiny step at a time. But, there has been a major change in the way those who are firmly entrenched within the world of traditional Western medicine view therapies generated by anyone outside their realm. In the early decades of the twentieth century, Western medicine doctors positively vilified other therapies and crusaded to make practicing other approaches illegal. In fact, well into the 1960s, talking to a chiropractor was considered unethical for a medical doctor!

Fortunately, the attitude that everything Western medical doctors do is great and other therapies are, by definition, evil, is falling by the wayside. As a society, we've learned that our medical doctors don't have the cures for all our ills, and that other approaches can offer a lot. But the alternative approaches aren't perfect. In fact, many alternate theories and practices aren't backed by enough scientific proof to be declared valid, and some things that alternative healers do have proven to be dangerous. Regardless of the debates surrounding these therapies, however, alternative medicine has become very popular. There are countless testimonials to the effectiveness of almost all types of alternative therapies, and a fair number of studies indicate that some of these approaches work as well as standard medicines — or even better.

Alternative Medicine and Its Monikers

Alternative, complementary, holistic, unorthodox, integrative, and preventive medicine: Many terms are used, often interchangeably. But what do they mean? Defining modern Western medicine (the drugs-and-surgery approach used by medical doctors) as *conventional medicine* is the first step in deciphering the many names of alternative medicine. Anything that's not conventional is considered *unorthodox medicine. Alternative medicine* is an approach used in place of conventional medicine, while *complementary medicine* works with conventional therapies. The concepts of *holistic* and *integrative medicine* are related to each other. Instead of focusing only on the symptoms or the damaged part of the body, the idea behind holistic and integrative medicine is to examine and treat the entire person, including the body, mind, emotions, and spirit. With *preventive medicine,* the goal is to close the door on disease and keep it from striking in the first place. Education, lifestyle changes, and buffing up the body, mind, emotions, and/or spirit are part of this preemptive campaign.

The most recent term used to describe alternative approaches to conventional medicine is *complementary and alternative medicine*, or CAM for short. According to the National Center for Complementary and Alternative Medicine, which is a part of the National Institutes of Health, CAM incorporates a variety of healing approaches that are, generally speaking, not taught in many medical schools, not used in many hospitals, and not covered by insurance companies.The mere fact that the National Institutes of Health has a division dedicated to complementary and alternative medicine means that acupuncture, massage, nutritional healing, herbology, chiropractic, and other therapies have finally gained a measure of popularity and recognition. Establishing the Center for Complementary and Alternative Medicine legitimized various therapies, and some money (not a lot, but some) is being spent to research these alternative and complementary therapies.

CAM is popular

Nearly half of all Americans have used at least one CAM at one time or another, and more than 80 million are expected to use CAM this year — sometimes to complement and sometimes to replace standard treatment. All told, Americans pay more visits to complementary and alternative healers than to primary medical doctors.

According to the *Los Angeles Times,* relaxation and herbs are the most popular CAM therapies.

Who sees CAM healers? Baby Boomers make up the largest chunk of patients, especially those who have graduated from college and earn more than $50,000 a year.

Another indication of the acceptance of complementary and alternative medicine is the fact that two-thirds of United States medical schools offer at least one course in complementary and alternative medicine. Most of these courses are electives (not required classes), but it's a start.

Finding a Reputable CAM Practitioner

You should select a CAM practitioner with the same care that you give to finding the right medical doctor. There are several ways to find the names of practitioners of various alternative forms of health care. You can find plenty of listings in the phone book. You can also get recommendations from friends or alternative healers that you're already seeing. The list of approved practitioners that your HMO or health insurance company may offer is another place to start your search. (Some HMOs and health insurance companies now pay for chiropractic or acupuncture services, and perhaps other forms of alternative care.) Likewise, you can get names of practitioners from the various societies to which they belong. (See the Resources section in this book for the names of some of these organizations.) Sometimes, asking your doctor or checking with your local hospital is also helpful, because a very small number of medical doctors practice one form of alternative medicine or another. Those who don't may make recommendations.

After you put together a list of possibilities, treat them just as you would a list of physicians you're considering. Ask them where they studied and whether they have a license or certification. Ask about their treatment philosophy. Ask what their treatment consists of, what it can do for you, what the side effects may be, how you know if the treatment is working, how the practitioner handles side effects, and so on. If you feel that your questions aren't answered forthrightly, or that you're being given the runaround, run out the door.

CAM practitioners may not perform surgery or inject you with drugs, but their actions can have serious consequences on your health.

Checking Credentials and Certifications

Complementary and alternative medicine has a lot to offer, and it can fill in some of the gaps in conventional medical care. Unfortunately, CAM suffers from a lack of standards and standardization. Herbs, for example, may vary greatly in purity and potency. Although some CAM healers are incredibly knowledgeable and skillful, others are not.

Before selecting a complementary or alternative healer, it's best to

✔ **See a physician (a medical doctor) to get an accurate diagnosis.** Some forms of arthritis are easy to recognize; others are not. It's best to know exactly what you're dealing with before undergoing any kind of treatment, conventional or CAM.

✔ **Educate yourself.** Gather and study all the information you can about any given CAM therapy before subjecting yourself to it. Read books and articles, get information from the Internet, talk to people, and contact the professional organizations associated with the particular CAM that interests you. But remember: Take all the information that you gather with a grain of salt. Consider the source of the information carefully. Is the person or group that offers this information knowledgeable? Does he or she have a solid educational background and/or practical experience? Is he or she an unbiased source or a salesperson?

✔ **Ask for credentials.** Ask the CAM therapist where he or she studied, if he or she is licensed by the state, certified by a board, and so on. Don't be shy or afraid to ask questions. Any healer — conventional or CAM — who won't happily review his or her background with you isn't a good prospect. And don't be afraid to ask for the name and phone number of the school or society that issued their credentials and to investigate that organization.

✔ **Ask for references.** Ask the CAM therapist for the names and phone numbers of people he has already worked with. Contact these people; ask them what they were suffering from, what the CAM practitioner did for them, how well the therapy worked, what the side effects were (if any), and so on.

✔ **Ask about the price.** Insurance does not cover most CAM therapies.

Identifying False Claims

Everyone wants a miracle pill that will cure his or her ills. And, everyone would like it even better if that pill was tiny and easy to swallow, worked instantly, didn't cost more than a pack of bubble gum, and only had to be taken once.

Unfortunately, such a cure doesn't yet exist for arthritis. This fact hasn't stopped some people from claiming that they have miracle cures for all your aches and pains, however. Most alternative practitioners are honest and sincere, but there are always hucksters who will happily tell you tales to take your money. So safeguard your health and pocketbook by watching for the following warning signs.

The secret formula trap

Be wary if the cure offers no list of ingredients or is based on a secret formula. Claiming that something is made from a secret formula can be an easy way for hucksters to avoid admitting that their "cure" doesn't contain anything remarkable. Reputable healers, on the other hand, are happy to tell you exactly what they're proposing that you take. And it's important that you know what you're taking, for even if the stuff in the "secret formula" is helpful, it may interact dangerously with a medicine or supplement you're taking. Or perhaps you're allergic to the secret stuff, or it's just not right for you.

Cites only one study

Proceed with caution if the health practitioner bases all the claims for the treatment on only one study. It's true that one study may be all that's needed to establish that a treatment works, but it's better if the therapy has been studied many times, with different patients and under different conditions. A therapy may work in one study with, say, elderly and bedridden osteoarthritis patients, but not work so well when tested again with younger or more active subjects. The more studies, the better. Reputable healers know this, which is why they want to cite as many studies as possible for their therapies.

Works for all types of arthritis

Avoid cures that purport to work for all types of arthritis — and other diseases as well. Nothing is a cure-all. As you recall from the discussion of arthritis early in this book, the many different forms have widely different causes and symptoms. How could one remedy work for all of them?

Cites only case histories

Be wary of any therapy if its proof of effectiveness is made up entirely of case histories. Although the case histories may be absolutely genuine, they aren't as valid as large scale, long term, carefully controlled scientific studies. After all, the patients in the case histories may not have had the same form of arthritis as you do, may have had complicating conditions, and may not have been given uniform doses of the therapy. There's also the possibility that the placebo effect accounts for the good results in the case histories. (That is, some of the patients may have gotten better primarily because they believed in the therapy.) Remember, however, that a lack of studies doesn't mean that a therapy is bad, and good study results by themselves do not guarantee that a treatment or therapy will work for you. Having a combination of both studies and case histories to review is best.

The miracle cure trap

Steer clear of practitioners who promise that their approach is the long-awaited miracle cure, the magic potion that will magically erase all your problems. Some standard and alternative cures are amazingly effective, but no one has yet developed the miracle cure that eases all our ills.

Shady demands from practitioners

Avoid practitioners who tell you to throw away your crutches, stop taking your medicine, and/or ignore your physician's advice. Likewise, be wary of practitioners who demand large amounts of money in advance, as well as those who don't want you to tell your physician what they're doing for you.

Working with Your Doctor

At least 40 percent of patients use alternative therapies, but perhaps three-quarters of them don't tell their physicians what they're doing. Many patients don't inform their physicians, because they're afraid that their doctors will pooh-pooh their ideas, tell them that they're foolish, try to talk them out of it, or even refuse to continue working with them if they insist on using CAM.

You, too, may be tempted to keep what you're doing a secret from your physician, but don't. Telling your physician everything you're doing, from taking vitamins or the "deep enemas" called colonics to undergoing chiropractic care or acupuncture, is important, because you may inadvertently be doing something that can harm you. Or, your physician may unknowingly prescribe a drug that clashes with something else you're taking.

Talking to physicians about alternatives can be difficult. They have the weight of medical authority on their side. They've gone to medical school and can speak a language that you may not understand. But don't be intimidated. Doctors work for you; they're here to serve you. You have the right to ask questions and receive complete answers. To practice medicine effectively, a doctor must also practice good communication. A physician who closes his or her ears tosses away an important tool. Here are some tips to help you discuss CAM with your physician:

 ✔ **Begin with the assumption that your physician will be supportive.** If you open your conversation with a challenge or disparaging remark, you probably won't get very far. Make it clear up front that you're not challenging or rejecting your doctor's ideas, but that you're simply looking for more information and help.

✔ **Ask your physician what he or she knows about the CAM in which you're interested.** Ask your physician if the CAM is appropriate for your ailment, if you need to watch out for anything while participating in the alternative therapy, and so on.

✔ **If your physician doesn't know about the CAM that interests you, offer him or her information.** Go online and get studies about the CAM, copy pages from articles and books, ask the CAM's professional organizations to supply you with information, and then help your doctor learn about the CAM that you're considering.

✔ **If there's not time to discuss CAM during this visit, ask for another appointment.** Offer to pay for the extra appointment, if necessary.

✔ **If your physician gives you trouble, ask why.** Does he or she know that this CAM is dangerous? Has he or she had a bad experience with it? Has he or she seen patients for which the CAM had negative or dangerous results? Is his or her objection based on knowledge or simply a feeling that anything unconventional is bad?

✔ **If your physician refuses to discuss CAM with you and/or refuses to work with you if you're using a CAM, get a new doctor.** Closed-mindedness is a terrible trait in any healer and may limit your road to recovery.

The Arthritis Foundation reports that female physicians are more open to CAM and are more likely to initiate a discussion and make suggestions on alternatives than their male counterparts.

Be as open-minded as you want your physician to be. Keep your mind open to hearing bad reports about the CAM that interests you, as well as good reports. No healing art, conventional or unconventional, is perfect. Each has its strengths and weaknesses, and it's best to know what your CAM can do for you — and what it can't.

Chapter 16

Herbs and Homeopathy

· ·

In This Chapter

▶ Knowing the difference between herbs and drugs

▶ Treating arthritis with herbs

▶ Finding out what homeopathy is and how it works

▶ Combating arthritis with homeopathic remedies

· ·

*E*ver since man began to roam the earth, healers have been using herbs — the roots, bark, stems, leaves, and any other part of certain plants — to cure or at least alleviate whatever ails us. Some herbs are eaten in their natural form; others are ground into powder, crushed or squeezed to make oil or extract, brewed with boiling water to make tea, and/or mixed with beeswax, petroleum jelly, or cream to make ointment or balm.

What's the difference between a healing herb and a drug? Drugs are often stripped, highly refined versions of herbs. About one quarter of all our modern medicines come from herbs. To turn an herb into a drug, pharmacological researchers work with the herb, refining it and homing in on the main ingredient. This ingredient is separated from the rest of the plant, modified in some way, perhaps concentrated, and standardized so that each pill or capsule delivers an exact amount. Then it's sold as a drug.

The good part about this approach is that it allows us to extract the special part of the herb, like a great soloist in an orchestra, that cures a particular ill. The bad part is that it only lets us have that soloist, while casting aside the rest of the orchestra.

Modern medicine favors the soloists, insisting that the rest of the orchestra is distracting, irrelevant, inferior, and/or counterproductive. Herbalists, on the other hand, argue that the sweetest music is made by many. The violin may carry the melody line, but all the other instruments are necessary to support, enhance, punctuate, and sweeten the sound. Is a soloist better than a full orchestra? The answer depends upon your perspective and needs.

Doctors say drugs are better because the active ingredient is isolated, they're modified and pure, they're served up strong, and they work much faster than herbs.

Herbs — everything old is new again!

No one knows exactly when man began using herbs or who realized that eating certain leaves could help stop an ache in the head and that drinking the liquid made from boiling roots in water could bring on sleep. But once the connection was made, people undoubtedly gathered whatever they could find and started experimenting. Some worked well and others sent them back to the drawing board. Herbs were a vital part of ancient medicine. The Egyptians used garlic and other herbs as medicines as early as 1800 B.C. Hippocrates, the Greek who fathered modern medicine, developed a way to classify herbs based on qualities such as heat versus coldness, and dampness and dryness. Herbs were the backbone of medicine until the development of modern medicine in the 19th and 20th centuries, and continue to be a mainstay of Native American, Ayurvedic, and Oriental medicines.

Although herbs, like homeopathic remedies and other therapies, were swept aside by the tidal wave of pharmaceutical drugs pouring out of laboratories during the 20th century, they were certainly never forgotten. Indeed, they still serve as the source of one-fifth of all modern drugs. Even today, pharmaceutical companies are scouring the world (especially the tropical rainforests), looking for previously unknown plants that that may have medicinal prowess. They also routinely ask herbalists and traditional healers about herbs in their quest for new sources of drugs.

Herbalists say that herbs are better because the so-called active ingredient is only one of many substances that work in concert to relieve or cure ailments. Modifying and purifying the active ingredients makes them overly strong, dangerous, and likely to cause side effects. Herbalists point out that some of the alleged impurities in herbs can actually make them gentler, thus safer. And while speed is sometimes necessary, many times it's not. Furthermore, drugs that work fast tend to hit too hard.

It's certainly true that most drugs are more potent and potentially dangerous than most herbs. Bear in mind, however, that while herbs are generally considered safer and gentler than drugs, some can pack quite a punch. The fact that something is natural does not guarantee that it's safe — think of arsenic.

Herbs for Arthritis

Which herbs have medicinal value? How much should be used? Which are good for osteoarthritis, which for rheumatoid arthritis and gout? Should they be taken in powder form, rubbed on as ointment, or sipped in the form of tea? The answers you get to these and many other herbal questions may depend on whom you ask, and whether he is a Doctor of Oriental Medicine, an herbologist, a naturopath, a chiropractor, or the clerk at the vitamin store.

Unfortunately, there is no national board of herbology to set standards and dosages, so the advice you receive about herbs to treat arthritis will undoubtedly vary from one healer to another. A variety of herbs may be prescribed, some specifically for your type of arthritis, others for joint problems in general, and still others for pain, depression, and/or strengthening the immune system.

Even though many people consider herbs to be safe, it's best not to self-medicate. You could do more harm than good to yourself, especially under the following circumstances:

- ✔ You may have a bad reaction.
- ✔ The herb may interact with a medicine that you're taking.
- ✔ You may have a condition that makes it dangerous for you to take a particular herb.
- ✔ The herbal concentration is too strong, too weak, or the herb is mixed with other ingredients that your body cannot handle.

That's why it's best to check with your health advisor before taking any herbs. Make sure your physician knows that you are taking herbs or planning to take them. Even if he is not an advocate of alternative healing methods, your physician should be aware of everything you're taking.

Inside the herbalist's toolbox . . .

Herbal medicine has been used to treat just about anything that can go wrong with the human body. There's a tremendous number of herbs in the herbalist's little black bag, including:

- ✔ *Agrimony* for allergies
- ✔ *Cayenne pepper* to strengthen the immune system
- ✔ *Celery* for arthritis
- ✔ *Feverfew* for migraine headaches
- ✔ *Fringe tree bark* for liver disease
- ✔ *Garlic* for elevated cholesterol and blood pressure
- ✔ *Ginger* for nausea
- ✔ *Ginkgo biloba* for problems with memory and circulation

- ✔ *Goto kola* for varicose veins
- ✔ *Hemp* for glaucoma
- ✔ *Hyssop* for asthma
- ✔ *Kava kava* for anxiety and insomnia
- ✔ *Linden* for tension
- ✔ *Sambucol,* an elderberry extract, for the flu
- ✔ *Skullcap* for asthma
- ✔ *St. John's wort* for insomnia and depression
- ✔ *Turmeric* for inflammation
- ✔ *Valerian* for asthma
- ✔ *Vervian* for headaches

Tea, please

Not all herbs are taken as pills or capsules. Some are taken in the form of teas or, more correctly, "infusions." (Technically speaking, the only true "tea" is one made from tea leaves, or the leaves of the *Camellia sinensis* bush.) To make an infusion, the herb is submerged in water that is just slightly cooler than boiling, then left to steep as its health-promoting ingredients seep into the water. After a few minutes, the herb is skimmed out, and the liquid is ready for drinking.

Try these infusions, as they suit your mood:

- ✔ **For a "pick me up"**: Basil, borage, ginseng, Hawthorne berry, bilberry, cinnamon, yarrow

- ✔ **For depression, stress or tension**: Borage, catnip, jasmine, hops

- ✔ **To strengthen the immune system**: Elderflower, green tea, goldenseal

- ✔ **For a digestive aid**: Ginger, juniper berry, Iceland moss, alfalfa, angelica

- ✔ **To promote sleep**: Chamomile, orange flower, valerian

Anti-inflammatories

Inflammation is a major problem in several forms of arthritis and related conditions. Doctors have powerful anti-inflammatory drugs, but many people prefer the gentle relief offered by herbs. Anti-inflammatory herbs don't suppress inflammation on their own as much as they help the body reduce the inflammation naturally.

Alfalfa

Rich in minerals, alfalfa is a folk remedy for arthritis favored in the Middle East for its ability to reduce swelling and inflammation. Alfalfa is scientifically known as *Medicago sativa*.

Angelica

Angelica, or *Angelica archangelica,* has been used treat the inflammation associated with rheumatism. This herb is also believed to purify the blood and protect against contagious diseases.

Black cohosh

Scientifically known as *Cimicifuga racemosa,* black cohosh is a Native American remedy taken to reduce the inflammation and pain of rheumatoid arthritis.

Bladderwrack

First coming into prominence in the early 1800s, Bladderwrack was originally used as a source of iodine. Today the herb, known by the scientific name of *Fucus vesiculosus,* is used in compresses to help reduce arthritis inflammation.

Boswellia

Known scientifically as *Boswellia serata,* boswellia comes from India, where its gummy resin has been used for thousands of years as an anti-inflammatory. Substances in boswellia, called *boswellic acids,* are believed to reduce inflammation and help relieve the pain of osteoarthritis and rheumatoid arthritis. That's undoubtedly why the herb has long been used in Ayurvedic medicine to treat arthritis and musculoskeletal pain. It has also been used to treat psoriasis, ulcerative colitis, and allergies, and may also help lower high cholesterol and high triglyceride levels. Boswellia is used as an extract, cream or ointment.

Cat's claw

The extract of the bark of a vine native to the Peruvian rainforest, cat's claw was used for generations by the Ashanica Indians of South America to treat colds, tumors, and cold sores. Known scientifically as *Uncaria tomentosa,* the herb is felt to be useful in combating arthritis symptoms in several ways. It may be recommended by herbalists to reduce inflammation, boost the immune system, and ward off free radical damage to the cells. Cat's claw is taken in the form of tea or capsules. The herb may also help counteract gastrointestinal damage caused by NSAIDs.

Centaury

Also known by it's scientific name, *Erythrina centaurium,* centaury was used by the ancient Egyptians to reduce high blood pressure, and later by German herbalists for anxiety and melancholy. Today, it's often recommended for cases of gout and rheumatism because of its ability to help relieve inflammation.

Devil's claw

Devil's Claw, or *Harpagophytum procumbens,* is the root of an herb grown in Africa. An infusion made of devil's claw, which is felt to reduce joint inflammation and pain, is a folk remedy for arthritis, rheumatism, and gout. This herb is most commonly used in capsule, tea, and tincture form. Devil's claw contains harpagoside, which has pain relieving and inflammation reducing qualities that have been compared to cortisone and phenylbutazone.

Sarsaparilla

With the official name of *Smilax officinalis,* sarsaparilla originated in the New World and was brought to Europe in the 1600s. There, the herb was used to treat inflammation due to rheumatoid arthritis. Herbalists still use it today to relieve the pain and swelling of arthritis and to enhance overall well being.

Wild yam

Known scientifically as *Dioscorea villosa,* wild yam is perhaps most famous as a traditional "female remedy," used for menstrual ailments and to prevent miscarriage. It also has anti-inflammatory properties, which is why herbalists recommend it for rheumatoid and other forms of inflammatory arthritis.

Antirheumatics

Several herbs seem to be especially helpful in reducing the symptoms of rheumatoid arthritis and related conditions. Here are a few of better-known antirheumatics.

Bogbean

Once used to prevent scurvy, this pretty wildflower is renowned for its ability to relieve the pain of rheumatism. Known to scientists as *Menyanthes trifoliate*, is has mild sedative properties.

Be careful, however, for large doses may cause vomiting. It should not be used if you have inflammatory bowel disease.

Celery Seed

Scientifically known as *Apium graveolens,* celery seed was used by Oriental healers to reduce elevated blood pressure. And the celery stalk was prized by Americans during the 1800s because it was so expensive. Today, celery seed and celery juice are used to rid the body of excess water and aid in digestion. The seed is also believed to ease both rheumatoid arthritis and gout.

Meadowsweet

Meadowsweet *(Filipendula ulmaria)* contains a substance with aspirin-like properties. The herb has been used for hundreds of years to relieve arthritis pain and help combat rheumatic conditions.

Sedatives and muscle relaxants

Sleep can be a major issue for those with some forms of arthritis. How well can you sleep if you hurt, if movement is difficult, or if you're worried and stressed? The herbs in this category can help you relax and sleep better.

Kava kava

A popular treatment for insomnia and nervousness, kava kava *(Piper methysticum)* promotes relaxation of the muscles and nervous system without diminishing mental alertness. By helping you relax and perhaps sleep better, this herb can help you deal more effectively with the stress of arthritis.

Valerian

Known as *Valeriana officinalis,* valerian comes from the rootstock or roots of a perennial herb. It is typically used in the form of capsules and extracts. Valerian is recommended for arthritis patients because it helps ease pain and tension, and it also encourages sleep. In Germany, valerian is used as a mild sedative, and one study showed that it worked as well as a standard sedative, drug with the added advantage of being non-addictive.

Don't take more than the recommended dosage — very high doses can cause a weakened heartbeat and even paralysis. Check with your physician to see how much you should take.

Pain relievers

Pain is perhaps the most significant symptom of many forms of arthritis. Dull or sharp, constant or intermittent, achey or gripping, pain can make your life miserable. Here are some of the better-known herbs that can help relieve pain.

Aloe

Used internally or externally, aloe is a popular herbal cure for the pain of wounds, burns, and arthritis. Known to the scientific community as *Aloe vera* or *Aloe barbadenis,* it can also be used in many forms: as a fresh leaf, a gel, capsule, lotion, and liquid. In addition to relieving arthritis pain, it has been used to treat gastrointestinal problems and ulcers, as first aid for wounds and burns, and as a mild laxative.

Taken internally, aloe may hamper the action of certain medications.

Burdock

Burdock *(Arctium lappa)* is an ancient remedy that has been used to treat snakebites, dog bites, and a variety of other conditions thought to leave impurities in the blood. Today's herbalists have found that burdock has a diuretic effect and may ease arthritis pain, as well as skin irritation due to psoriasis, eczema, and canker sores.

Capsaicin

Capsaicin, which comes from chili peppers, is the ingredient in the spice cayenne that makes it "hot." Capsaicin is believed to prompt the release of endorphins, the body's natural, built-in pain relievers, and to interfere with substance P, which helps transmit nerve signals through the nervous system. Known scientifically as *Capsicum frutescens,* capsaicin is used to treat pain. It's typically applied as a cream or taken as a tea or capsule.

Fennel

Well-known among chefs, fennel has been used to relieve stiff, painful joints. Herbalists and folk medicine healers often suggest that their patients apply fennel oil directly to their distressed joints and rub it in. This herb's scientific name is *Foeniculum vulgare.*

Ginger

The aromatic root of a tropical herb, ginger has been used by the Chinese to treat indigestion, stomach cramps, and stomach upset for over 2,000 years. Scientifically known as *Zingiber officinale,* ginger may be recommended for arthritis patients by modern herbalists. Studies have shown that taking ginger supplements or eating fresh ginger can help ease the pain, morning stiffness, and inflammation associated with some forms of arthritis, while increasing flexibility and range-of-motion.

Ginger is typically taken as a powder, capsule, extract, tea, or as a tincture. It can also be freshly grated and added to food or eaten as a side dish. Ginger compresses may be applied to painful joints.

Mustard (black)

A preparation of mustard, or *Brassica nigra*, has long been a favorite remedy for painful joints. Sometimes it's taken internally — often with honey — and sometimes it's applied directly to the joint. (Mustard oil plus rubbing alcohol can be applied to the skin to increase circulation to the affected area.) Black mustard is generally considered stronger and more effective than white mustard.

Stinging nettle

A prickly plant with stinging hairs that "inject" an irritant into the skin, stinging nettle has traditionally been used to treat allergies, insect bites, and wounds. Today it may be recommended to relieve joint pain and swelling, because laboratory studies suggest that stinging nettle can counteract at least some part of the inflammatory response. A German study found stinging nettle plus a small amount of an NSAID to be as effective as the full dose of the NSAID in relieving symptoms of osteoarthritis. In addition, stinging nettle contains boron, a mineral important for bone health. Known scientifically as *Urtica dioica,* stinging nettle is typically taken as a capsule or extract. A poultice of cooked leaves may be applied to the painful area.

Besides the preceding herbs, your herbalist may suggest black willow, caraway seed, cinnamon, clove, couchgrass, dandelion, juniper berries, oats, nutmeg, poke root, prickly ash, skullcap, spearmint, star anise, wintergreen, wormwood, yarrow, and more. Suffice it to say, there's a lengthy list of herbs that an herbalist may recommend for arthritis pain, inflammation, anxiety, depression, insomnia, skin rashes, muscle pains, and other symptoms!

Herbal definitions

A lot of terms are casually tossed about by herbalists and herbal enthusiasts: extract, infusion, and so on. Here are a few definitions to help you find your way through the sometimes-confusing world of "herbal speak."

✔ **Extract:** A key ingredient of an herb or plant is isolated and drawn out, using steam or water, then condensed into liquid or powder form, known as an extract.

✔ **Herb:** A plant or part of a plant valued for its medicinal, aromatic, or savory qualities.

✔ **Infusion:** Boiling water is poured over an herb or plant part, then allowed to steep to release the plant's useful qualities into the liquid.

✔ **Raw herbs:** Fresh or dried parts of plants, plucked right from the ground, bush, vine, or tree.

✔ **Standardized extract:** An herbal extract manufactured to deliver an exact concentration of the desired ingredient.

✔ **Tincture:** Herbal preparations made by steeping herbs in alcohol.

Homeopathy: Like Cures Like

Before drugs and surgery came to dominate Western medicine, healers called *homeopaths* flourished in the United States and Europe. Their guiding philosophy was *homeopathy*, which means "similar suffering."

The idea behind homeopathy, which was created by Dr. Samuel Hahnemann in the eighteenth century, is to stimulate the body's natural healing mechanisms by, in a sense, "showing" it a piece of what's wrong. This may sound odd; after all, we're accustomed to modern Western medicine killing disease with strong medicines. But Dr. Hahnemann believed that "like cures like." If large amounts of a substance could cause the symptoms of a disease in a healthy person, he reasoned, then very small amounts of the same substance should be able to help the body eliminate the same ailment. These small doses would act something like vaccines and gently stimulate the body to heal itself.

For example, suppose that a large amount of Substance X caused constipation in healthy people. According to Dr. Hahnemann's homeopathic theory, a very tiny dose of the same Substance X would unlock the bowels in people who were already constipated. This idea was codified as homeopathy's *Law of Similars*.

Your symptoms determine the remedies

While medical doctors try to suppress symptoms, doctors of homeopathy look upon them as helpful signs that the body is trying to heal itself. To the homeopath, symptoms are more than simply indicators that a certain disease is present. Instead, they are the body's way of describing what has gone wrong on a physical, mental, and emotional level. Probing beyond the symptoms (where Western medicine stops), homeopaths look for the essence of their patients. Thus, they'll ask what the patients like to eat and drink, when and how well they sleep, whether they're day or night people, what they wish for and what they fear, what kind of weather they prefer, how they respond to stress, and so on.

If you complain of pain, a good homeopath will look beyond its location, intensity, and number of occurrences. He or she will ask additional questions, such as:

- When does it hurt?
- What are you doing when it starts to hurt?
- How are you feeling, emotionally, before the pain strikes?
- What does the pain feel like? Is it sharp? Throbbing? An ache? Does it radiate? Is it constant? Does it come and go?
- What makes the pain feel better? A warm bath? Eating certain foods? Going to work?
- What makes it feel worse? Movement? Cold temperatures? Stress? Work? Family gatherings? Holidays?

These kinds of questions are designed to get to the essence of the problem, the physical and emotional state that allowed the disease to take hold and grow.

After the homeopath identifies the essential problem, it can be treated — but not with a medicine designed to destroy anything. Instead, the homeopath looks for the single best remedy (homeopathic "medicine.") What remedy is most effective depends mostly on the patient. If a patient has joint pain, for example, not just any remedy for pain will do. It has to be the remedy that best matches the patient's *constitutional makeup*. Every one of the 2,000 or so homeopathic remedies closely matches a particular temperament — a person's fears and hopes, likes and dislikes, and sleep and behavior patterns.

In *classical homeopathy,* only the absolute minimum dose of a remedy is given, and only one remedy is prescribed at a time. If the right remedy is given, the patient's symptoms will begin to clear up in a few days. If not, a different remedy is selected. No new remedies are used after the body has begun to heal itself. Practitioners of *complex homeopathy,* however, *will* prescribe more than one remedy at a time.

Homeopathic remedies for arthritis

Most homeopathic remedies come from minerals or plants, with only a few derived from animals. Homeopathic remedies are not highly concentrated; in fact, they're diluted again and again until only minuscule amounts of the original substance are left.

This method is counter-intuitive to practitioners of Western medicine, who believe that medicines should have more of the active ingredient, not less. But remember, homeopaths argue that smaller portions are better, because larger portions can cause the arthritic problem. It's the tiny portions, they insist, that help the body heal itself.

Shaken, not stirred

The 2,000 or so homeopathic remedies are derived for a variety of sources: leaves, berries, fruits, bark, roots, minerals and sometimes animals. But no matter where they come from, they're all processed in a very special way.

In keeping with the idea that small amounts are best, the remedies are diluted over and over again in solutions made of water and alcohol, lactose, or other diluents. And each time they're diluted, they are shaken and struck in a special way. The more diluted, shaken, and struck, so the theory goes, the stronger the remedy becomes. Indeed, a finished remedy may only contain one part per million of the active ingredient. Critics charge that there's very little or even none of the active ingredient remaining after these successive dilutions, so the remedy couldn't possibly work. Supporters believe that either 1) what's left over is enough to do the trick; or 2) that the fluid retains a "molecular memory" of the medicinal substance and acts accordingly.

Remedies are rated according to their potency. When one drop of the medicinal substance is shaken and struck into 99 drops of diluent, the remedy has a potency rating of 1c. (This is sometimes written as 1CH.) If one drop is taken out of this mixture and added to 99 drops of new diluent, the new remedy has a potency rating of 2c. If one drop of the 2c remedy is then diluted with 99 drops of a new diluent, the potency rating rises to 3c, and so on.

How potent the remedy should be depends on the state of the disease. Here are the general guidelines used in the U.S. and many other countries:

- **Low potency:** Up to 6c, used when there are only physical symptoms or severe changes in the disease state.

- **Medium potency:** From 12-30c, used when there are physical and mental/emotional symptoms.

- **High potency:** Up to 200c or greater, used when the problem is long-standing or acute, or the symptoms are mental/emotional.

There's another, very similar rating system based on 10 drops of diluent rather than 99. Instead of shaking and striking one drop of substance into 99 drops of diluent, you use only 9 drops of diluent. In this method, based on ten drops, potencies are rated 1x (or D), 2x, 3x, and so on.

It's never a good idea to self-medicate. No matter how much you may have heard about the safety of homeopathic remedies, it's essential that you work with a medical doctor or doctor of homeopathy when using them. If you are using any homeopathic remedies, be sure your physician knows exactly what and how much you're taking. Even if he or she doesn't believe in homeopathy, your physician should be aware of what you're taking.

The purpose of the homeopath is to find the best match between remedy and patient. Remember: The remedy that the homeopath selects depends as much on the patient's constitutional makeup as it does on the symptoms, which is why you can't just pull any old arthritis remedy off the shelf. The following are some of the homeopathic remedies used for arthritis:

- ✔ **Actea spic:** May be indicated when the joints are swollen and pained, and the focus of the arthritis is in the hands and feet or the smaller joints.

- ✔ **Aconitum napellus:** May be indicated for gout. The pain grows worse at night or when temperatures rise, and gets better when the patient rests or gets fresh air. The patient is anxious and imagines terrible things are happening.

- ✔ **Ammonium carbonicum:** May be indicated when there is poor circulation to the hands, as in Raynaud's syndrome.

- ✔ **Apis mellifica:** May be indicated when the joints are stiff and swollen, when pressure makes the pain worse, and when the skin over the swollen joints feels stretched and tight.

- ✔ **Arnica montana:** May be indicated when the patient has rheumatoid arthritis linked to cold and dampness, and soreness and bruising are problems. The patient is nervous and extremely sensitive, prefers to be alone, and denies that anything is wrong.

- ✔ **Belladonna:** May be indicated for sudden, sharp pain, and red, swollen joints. Getting wet or chilled makes the pain worse, and the patient usually avoids any kind of stimulation.

- ✔ **Benzoic acid:** May be indicated when rheumatoid arthritis settles in the smaller joints, and there are nodular swellings.

- ✔ **Bryonia alba:** May be indicated for gout with greatly swollen joints. Heat, movement, or touch makes the pain worse; cold, rest, and pressure help.

- ✔ **Calcarea carbonica-ostrearum:** May be indicated for rheumatoid arthritis in the shoulders and upper back. Wetness and dampness worsen the pain and fear and perhaps confusion engulfs the patient.

- ✔ **Causticum:** May be indicated when arthritic joints are stiff and tight. Lying on the afflicted joints increases the soreness, and the patient is restless at night.

✔ *Chamomilla:* May be indicated for severe pain when anger and restlessness are present.

✔ *Cimicifuga racemosa:* May be indicated when pain is centered more in the muscles than the bones. Restlessness, talkativeness, and an unstable mood often accompany the pain.

✔ *Ledum palustre:* May be indicated when pain is primarily in the smaller joints and travels up the body, with little or no swelling. Pain is worse when patient is in a warm bed.

✔ *Ruta graveolens:* May be indicated when the patient suffers from bursitis.

✔ *Sabina:* May be indicated when the patient is suffering from gout, and the gouty joints have nodules. The pain worsens with heat and movement, feels better with cool air, and is usually accompanied by depression.

✔ *Sambucus:* May be indicated when the patient is suffering from poor circulation to the hands, as in Raynaud's Syndrome. The hands are blue and cold and the patient sweats excessively while awake, but not while sleeping.

Finding Homeopathic Help

No one has proven why or how homeopathy may work, and while some studies suggest that it's significantly more effective than a placebo, others have found it unimpressive. Although all the evidence is not yet in, there are many people who are convinced that homeopathy is right for them. Homeopathy is practiced by a variety of healers in the United States: naturopaths, chiropractors, herbalists, dentists, acupuncturists, and even certain medical doctors and Doctors of Osteopathy (D.O.'s). The level of training and skill, however, will vary from healer to healer, so be forewarned!

The National Center for Homeopathy (see Appendix B: Resources) offers a directory of homeopaths in the United States. You can also find homeopaths by asking for referrals from certain physicians and other health professionals, reading the ads or listings in alternative health newspapers and magazines, or contacting homeopathic pharmacies.

Chapter 17

Hands-On Healing Methods

· ·

In This Chapter

▶ Exploring the different types of Eastern and Western touch therapies

▶ Understanding the theory behind the therapy

▶ Knowing what to expect during a therapy session

▶ Understanding the possible benefits of each therapy

▶ Finding a competent practitioner

· ·

*F*or thousands of years, healers have known that the "laying on of hands" can have a powerful therapeutic effect on the body. And why wouldn't it? Human beings are made to be touched: Babies fail to thrive if they're not touched enough. Huddling together against the cold was undoubtedly a survival technique for scores of our ancestors, and lovemaking is perhaps one of life's most fulfilling, restorative activities. Therefore, looking to hands-on methods for healing your body when it's ill or in pain makes sense. This will not necessarily cure the disease, but it can help relieve pain, increase vital circulation, ease mental stress, relax tensed muscles, increase overall relaxation, and to aid the body in its struggle to rebuild itself.

The various methods of "hands-on" therapy, from the ancient acupressure to the relatively new trigger point therapy, are explored in this chapter. Keep in mind, however, that if you decide to engage in any of these therapies, you should use them in addition to — not in place of — standard medical treatment, and you should first discuss your preferred therapy method with your physician.

Eastern "Hands-On" Healing Methods

These therapies, which are rooted in either Chinese or Japanese medicine, are designed to remove blockages in the body's energy flow and restore balance. Then the body can begin to heal itself.

Acupuncture

An important part of traditional Chinese medicine, *acupuncture* has been used for thousands of years to prevent and treat disease by balancing the body's energy flow.

In traditional Chinese medicine, disease is thought to be the result of an imbalance or blockage of energy or *chi* (pronounced "chee") in one or more parts of the body. (Air and food supply us with energy, while the stresses and strains of living diminish this energy.) Acupuncturists believe that manipulating specific points on the body can unblock the energy flow and restore the body's balance.

According to traditional Chinese medicine theory, energy flows through the body along invisible channels called *meridians*. There are twelve major meridians running through your body delivering energy and sustenance to your tissues, but these channels can become obstructed. When they do, the obstructions act like tiny dams, blocking or slowing the flow of energy, which is believed to be a major cause of pain and disease. Luckily, the meridians touch the surface of your skin at some 300 different points called *acupuncture points*, and by manipulating and stimulating these points, the acupuncturist can remove the obstructions and reestablish the healthy flow of chi throughout your body.

When you first visit an acupuncturist, he or she will probably interview you extensively about your symptoms, level of pain, medical history, diet, bowel habits, quality of sleep, and so on. He or she may also examine your eyes, tongue, skin, or fingernails, take your pulse, and listen to your voice, breathing, and bowel sounds.

During your visit, you'll either lie or sit on a padded table for the treatment, but you won't have to remove all your clothing, just loosen it and uncover the areas to be treated. Your acupuncturist will then stimulate and manipulate certain acupressure points, but just a few, not all 300 of them! The following list explains the various methods your acupuncturist may use to stimulate and manipulate your acupuncture points.

> ✔ **Insertion of fine needles:** Your acupuncturist may insert anywhere from 2 to 15 hair-thin needles into certain points and leave them standing for a period of time (usually 20 to 40 minutes). He or she won't necessarily insert the needles directly into the area that's bothering you, but rather along the meridian that affects that area. So don't be surprised if your feet are manipulated to ease your back or neck pain! The needles are so fine, you may not feel them, but if you do, you usually feel just a moderate sting that disappears quickly. Your acupuncturist may insert needles just under your skin or as deep as an inch or more.

✔ **Insertion of fine needles connected to a low-level current (electro-acupuncture):** Many acupuncturists have found that the addition of a low-level electrical current can make the treatment more powerful. Wires are attached to the acupuncture needles after the needles are inserted, and these wires are hooked up to a box that delivers an electrical current. Your acupuncturist will adjust this current by turning a dial.You should feel a light buzzing at your acupuncture points. If the buzz is annoying or uncomfortable, tell your acupuncturist, and he or she will turn down the "juice" until it no longer bothers you.

✔ **Use of heat and herbs (moxibustion):** To stimulate your acupuncture points, your acupuncturist may burn a small amount of an herb called *mugwort* (or *moxa* in Chinese) over your acupuncture points, being careful not to burn your skin.

✔ **Cupping:** Small glass cups are heated and placed over your acupuncture points where they create a vacuum-like effect. As they cool, the cups invigorate these areas.

What can acupuncture do for me?

More than 15 million Americans have used acupuncture to treat ailments ranging from asthma to ulcers, but its primary use is for pain relief. Many people with osteoarthritis, rheumatoid arthritis, gout, fibromyalgia, and Raynaud's phenomenon swear by acupuncture, and some studies have shown that it can relieve pain due to osteoarthritis and/or fibromyalgia. Although there is no scientific explanation for its effectiveness, acupuncture does cause real responses in the body, including stimulation of the immune and circulatory systems and the release of endorphins, the body's natural painkillers.

You may require several acupuncture sessions (perhaps as many as six) before you begin to notice a difference, but once the beneficial effects set in, they often last for weeks, months, or even longer. Unfortunately, acupuncture doesn't work for everyone.

How can I find a good acupuncturist?

To find a good acupuncturist, begin looking for one who is licensed by the state, if your state happens to be one that licenses acupuncturists. (Some states don't.) It's also a good idea to look for a practitioner certified by The National Certification Commission for Acupuncture and Oriental Medicine (NCCAOM), acupuncture's equivalent to the American Medical Association. Some 9,000 practitioners have been certified by the NCCAOM, so you can probably find at least one in your area. Or, if you like the idea of receiving acupuncture from someone with a medical degree, contact the American Academy of Medical Acupuncture. They can provide you with a list of M.D.s or D.O.s (doctors of osteopathy) who have completed at least 220 hours of acupuncture training. (See "Acupuncture/Acupressure" in Appendix B for more information.)

Finally, ask the members of your health care team for referrals, as more members of the traditional Western medical community are becoming aware of the benefits of acupuncture. (Who knows? Maybe some of them see acupuncturists themselves!) It doesn't hurt to ask, and your medical team members may be able to give you some good leads.

Acupressure (shiatsu)

Acupressure (which the Japanese call *shiatsu*) is a lot like acupuncture, but instead of needles, the therapist presses on your acupuncture points using the fingers, hands, or special tools to unblock your energy flow and restore balance. Because acupressure involves hands-on manipulation, it's often considered another form of massage instead of a version of acupuncture. Because it's actually a combination of these two methods, acupressure is often used by both acupuncturists and massage therapists.

Instead of lying on a padded table as you do during an acupuncture session, you will lie on a mat on the floor for better resistance against the pressure exerted during treatment. Using the thumbs, fingers, whole hand, elbows, or feet, the practitioner applies pressure and manipulates your body along meridians to improve your flow of *chi* (energy). He or she may also use tools, such as wooden rollers, balls, or pointers. As the practitioner works to unblock your *chi,* he will also work to transmit some of his own energy into your body. Your acupressure session may include stretching or other kinds of massage, and some practitioners will also give diet and lifestyle tips.

What can acupressure do for me?

Acupressure is designed to produce the same pain relieving and energizing results as acupuncture — without the needles, of course! Like massage, acupressure has a calming and soothing effect, and that alone may help ease some of your symptoms almost immediately. Although good studies demonstrating its effectiveness don't currently exist, acupressure does work for some people, and (when it's properly done) there are no obvious side effects. At the very least, your acupressure session should be a pleasant experience.

How can I find a good acupressurist?

Contact the National Certification Commission for Acupuncture and Oriental Medicine (NCCAOM), the certifying board, to find an acupressurist. (See "Acupuncture/Acupressure" in Appendix B for more information.)

Many massage therapists also use acupressure techniques. To find one that does, check out the American Massage Therapy Association (AMTA) Web site. (See "Massage" in Appendix B). At the top of the AMTA homepage, click "Find A Massage Therapist," scroll down to "Technique," and use the arrow key to find "Shitasu/Acupressure."

You may also find referrals through your health care team, rehab center, pain management center, or chiropractor.

Reiki

The word *reiki* (pronounced ray-kee) is a combination of two Japanese words — *rei*, meaning a Higher Intelligence or spiritual consciousness, and *ki* (or *chi* in Chinese) meaning the life force or energy that animates all plants and animals. Therefore, *Reiki* is a healing energy that is guided by a higher intelligence or a spiritual power.

The Reiki practitioner will administer the treatment by laying his hands on specific parts of your body and applying little or no pressure. (You will remain fully clothed.) He will then channel healing energy into you, which helps to relieve energy blockages and balance the life force within your body. This technique is sometimes used along with some form of massage. The basic principle of Reiki is that universal life energy, which creates and maintains all forms of life, can be channeled into a patient by the practitioner as a force for healing.

What can Reiki do for me?

Reiki enthusiasts say that Reiki can help ease the pain and other symptoms of virtually every kind of illness and injury, while increasing the effectiveness of all kinds of therapy. Although the practitioner may not actually touch the patient, those who have experienced Reiki say that they feel a glowing radiance flowing throughout their bodies after a 60 to 90 minute session. Stress reduction, relaxation, and an increased sense of well-being are typical benefits of a session.

How can I find a good Reiki practitioner?

Check out The International Center for Reiki Training Web site (see "Reiki" in Appendix B for more information). The Web site's link, "Reiki Net Resources," gives the names of both Reiki practitioners and Reiki teachers, should you want to learn to practice the art yourself.

Western "Hands-On" Healing Methods

While Eastern therapies are based on releasing energy blockages and restoring the "chi," Western therapies contain a potpourri of approaches, ranging from manipulating the alignment of the spine to applying pressure to specific points on the sole of the foot. Each is based on a different theory, and each takes a completely unique approach to pain relief.

Chiropractic

First introduced to the Western world in late 1800s by Daniel David Palmer, chiropractic is based on the belief that the body has the power to heal itself, and that power is concentrated in the central nervous system, extending from the brain down through the end of the spine. According to Palmer, disease is the result of the spinal vertebrae causing undue pressure on nearby nerves. This pressure interferes with the healthy functioning of the tissues or organs served by those nerves, causing disease or damage. According to the chiropractic theory, manipulating the spine to relieve nerve pressure can eliminate illness and restore health.

Misalignments in the spine that put pressure on the nerves are called *subluxations* and can be caused by injury, poor posture, stress, lack of exercise, or genetic problems, just to name a few. You won't necessarily be able to feel that you have a subluxation (they're often very minor imbalances), and you probably won't realize that a misalignment in your back could cause the pain in your kidney. That's why you visit the chiropractor. He or she can tell by touch or other simple tests where your spine is out of alignment, and then adjust it accordingly.

The chiropractor will ask you about the location, duration, intensity, and length of time you've been experiencing the pain, and if it seems appropriate, may take an X ray of the area.

After your X ray, you'll go to the adjustment room where you'll lie face down on a padded table. The chiropractor will feel along your spine looking for vertebra that are out of line, tension in the muscles, swelling, or any other abnormalities. Then, he or she may use a variety of methods to apply controlled, directed forces to your spine, including straight massage, acupressure, trigger point therapy, and myofascial release. All these methods fall into the category of *spinal manipulative therapy* (SMT) and aim to release stress, improve alignment, relieve pain, and improve function. Many chiropractors will also use a tool called an *activator* that resembles a tiny, rubber-tipped pogo stick. The activator delivers a precise, measurable force that, when applied to specific points on your body, helps adjust misalignments. And, of course, the chiropractor may "crack" your back or neck to relieve pressure within a given area of your spine.

What can chiropractic do for me?

Chiropractic can be a very effective treatment for acute lower-back pain, as well as a faster, better way to treat certain types of neck and back pain than standard Western medicine, massage, or acupuncture. Chiropractic may also be a useful way to treat headaches, muscle spasms, knee pain, and shoulder pain. It is also used occasionally to relieve pain in the hip, knee, or shoulder, although it doesn't usually work as well as it does in the neck and spine.

Manipulating already-damaged joints can make them worse. Consult your physician before trying chiropractic, and make sure you let your chiropractor know that you have arthritis.

How can I find a good chiropractor?

Begin your search for a chiropractor through referrals from friends, especially if you know someone who has been treated by several chiropractors over the years and can compare their strengths and weaknesses. Otherwise, contact the American Chiropractic Association (see *Chiropractors* in Appendix B for more information) for a referral list and start making trial visits. Many types of insurance now cover chiropractic if you go to one of their designated practitioners, so you may want to get a list from your insurance company. Once you've narrowed your choices, look for a chiropractor who:

- ✔ Has had experience in treating patients with your type of arthritis.

- ✔ Spends at least 20 minutes with you each session, performing hands-on work.

- ✔ Doesn't pressure you to buy vitamins or supplements.

- ✔ Doesn't rely on gadgets such as back massaging beds, infrared lamps, waterbeds, or vibrators.

- ✔ Takes few if any X rays.

- ✔ Performs myofascial release or some other soft-tissue massage before adjusting your spine.

You may need several treatments before you see a noticeable improvement. However, if you aren't getting results after five or six treatments, chiropractic (or your current chiropractor) may not be for you.

Massage

Massage is the manipulation of body tissues by rubbing, stroking, kneading, or tapping using the hands or other instruments such as rollers, balls, or pointers. For most kinds of massage, you'll lie on a padded table, wearing little or no clothing, and covered by a soft flannel sheet. Your body will remain covered by the sheet throughout the massage, except for the area that's actually receiving the treatment.

If you're uncomfortable with the idea of disrobing in front of the therapist, remember that you only need to take off enough clothing to reveal the areas that you want massaged. Keeping your underwear on is definitely okay! It's also possible to be massaged while sitting in a chair, completely clothed. (Sometimes this is done in the workplace.)

The therapist will ask you what kind of massage you'd like (invigorating, relaxing, and so on), if and where you're experiencing any pain, and how firm or soft a touch you'd prefer. If you like, the therapist may darken the room and play soft music during the massage. Oil or lotion (usually prewarmed) will be used so that the therapist's hands will glide over your skin without causing friction.

Speak up! It's not necessary to get a whole body massage unless that's what you want. If you just want work done on your neck, feet, and hands, for example, say so. And don't be afraid to give your therapist feedback during the massage: Tell him or her what's painful, what's soothing, what you'd like more or less of, what kind of pressure feels best, and so on. The therapist will adjust the technique and pressure accordingly. The whole point of massage is for you to relax and feel comfortable, so be clear about what you need.

There are many kinds of massage, but here is a list of some of the most popular:

- **Swedish massage:** Also known as *effleurage*, Swedish massage involves the gentle kneading and stroking of muscles, connective tissue, and skin using oils or lotions. Sometimes clapping or tapping movements are also used. Therapists can make this method of massage as gentle or as vigorous as you like. If you have fibromyalgia, rheumatoid arthritis, or another particularly painful form of arthritis, a gentle Swedish massage may be just what you need to help you relax.

- **Shiatsu:** Also known as acupressure. (See "Acupressure," earlier in this chapter.)

- **Deep tissue massage:** This method of massage involves the exertion of intense pressure to relieve chronic tension deep within the muscles. Using fingers, thumbs, and sometimes elbows, aching, knotted, or chronically tense muscles are slowly stroked across the grain to release tension and induce relaxation. Deep tissue massage can be painful and may cause soreness during and after the session. But if favoring your painful joints causes chronic tension to develop in other parts of your body, deep tissue massage may be a way to release the tension.

Make sure you consult your doctor before trying deep tissue massage.

- **Rolfing:** Rolfing was developed in the 1950s by Ida P. Rolf, a biochemist who learned about therapeutic bodywork when an osteopath successfully treated her for a respiratory problem. Dr. Rolf's treatment is based on the idea that both physical and psychological health are affected by the alignment of the body. If the body is out of line, poor physical, mental, and emotional health results.

To correct body misalignment, the Rolfing practitioner stretches and manipulates the thin membrane called the *fascia* that covers each bone, muscle, organ, nerve, and blood vessel. The fascia can become tight in response to stress, injury, or chronic misuse. To release this tightness, the practitioner uses his or her fingers, knuckles, or elbows to apply intense pressure. Administered in one-hour sessions once a week for ten weeks, Rolfing is uncomfortable at best; at worst, it's quite painful. But proponents of this method claim that it can produce marked improvement in muscle function and reduced strain on the joints. Combined with special breathing techniques, Rolfing may also help release the buried emotions that create chronic physical tension.

✔ **Myofascial release:** Myofascial release is a milder form of Rolfing, in which the practitioner applies gentle but steady pressure to the fascia to stretch it and release tension.

Rolfing and/or myofascial release may be too painful for many arthritis patients. Make sure to get your doctor's permission before trying out either of these kinds of massage.

✔ **Sports massage:** This form of massage is intended to ease soreness, assist in healing sports injuries such as sprains, strains, tendonitis, or muscle soreness, and prevent future injury. Like Swedish massage, sports massage involves kneading and stroking the muscles and connective tissue, with an emphasis on the areas of your body most affected by the sport (for example, the shoulder and arm of a baseball pitcher or the knees and legs of a football player). If you have an injury or an inflamed joint, make sure that your massage therapist is a qualified expert in this type of massage.

✔ **Trigger point therapy:** Using the fingers to apply prolonged, deep tissue pressure to specific points on knotted, painful muscles, trigger point therapy relieves tension and helps muscle relax. This therapy causes the pain sensors in the pinpointed area to "overload," so they'll either send fewer pain messages or stop sending them altogether. In some cases, trigger point therapy can be a helpful treatment for fibroymyalgia.

Trigger point therapy is a treatment that feels so good — when it stops! Let's say, for example, that you have chronic tension in your neck that you just can't seem to release. To perform trigger point therapy, your massage therapist or chiropractor will ask you to lie face down on a padded table, and will then proceed to apply intense thumb pressure to a specific point where your neck and shoulders meet. (Yes, it hurts!) Your therapist will maintain this pressure for a good 30 to 45 seconds (or as long as you can stand it), but once the pressure is released, your chronic neck tension should be gone (or at least, greatly reduced).

As with deep tissue massage, Rolfing, and myofascial release, you should check with your doctor before engaging in trigger point therapy.

Injured and/or inflamed joints should not be massaged directly, as injured tissue may be further damaged, and the increased circulation brought about by massage may make swelling worse.

What can massage do for me?

Like most kinds of "hands-on" therapy, massage can significantly affect your well-being — at least temporarily. A slower heart rate, increased endorphin levels, decreased pain levels, and improved relaxation are just a few of the positive results. Like a nice warm bath, a good massage can increase your circulation and then go two steps further. It helps your body clear away by-products of metabolism that can irritate nerve endings and eases pain by increasing your level of endorphins — the body's natural morphine.

Some types of massage may not be appropriate for your type of arthritis. Consult your doctor for guidelines before getting massage therapy, especially if you have rheumatoid arthritis, osteoarthritis, or ankylosing spondylitis. Also, avoid massage if you've got a fever or infection, if you're having an arthritis flare-up, or if you're coming down with an acute illness.

How can I find a good massage therapist?

Locating a skilled massage therapist who is experienced in treating clients with arthritis should be one of your top priorities. Fortunately, your physical therapist or doctor may be able to steer you to someone who fills this bill.

For a therapist who specializes in a particular type of massage, consult the Web site of the American Massage Therapy Association (see "Massage Therapists" in Appendix B for more information). At the top of the homepage, click "Find A Massage Therapist," scroll down to "Technique," and use the arrow key to find the type of massage that interests you. You soon get a list of every member of AMTA in the U.S. who performs that kind of massage.

You can also get referrals from the The National Certification Board for Therapeutic Massage and Bodywork Web site or from your health care team, rehab center, pain management center, or chiropractor.

But just as important as technical qualifications is the chemistry between you and your therapist. The sex of the therapist, in fact, is an issue for many people. If you feel a little strange about being massaged by a man, for example, you should automatically narrow your search to include women only. Remember, if you don't feel completely comfortable with the therapist you choose, you won't be able to enjoy all the benefits of massage. So shop around; you may want to try several therapists before deciding on one person. Keep in mind that many massage therapists come to your home with their massage tables and all the accoutrements in tow. All you have to do is pick up the phone!

Polarity therapy

Like traditional Eastern systems of healing, *polarity therapy* is based on the belief that the body contains energy systems that must remain balanced, because unbalanced or blocked energy leads to pain and disease. The aim of polarity therapy is to find these blockages and release them by using the hands to touch specific points on the body, which should help restore balance. Once that is achieved, the body should return to a healthy state.

During your first visit, the practitioner will interview you, observe your body and the way you move, and manually feel certain areas of your body to determine the location and degree of your energy blockages. The therapy itself involves touches that can vary from light to firm, but you will not have to disrobe, and the touching will involve your verbal feedback. A typical session will last from an hour to an hour and a half.

What can polarity therapy do for me?

Your polarity therapy practitioner will work to help you increase your awareness of *subtle energetic sensations*. For example, you may feel mild waves of energy coursing through your body, tingling, warmth, or general relaxation. Your practitioner may also offer advice on diet and lifestyle. The idea is to relieve your pain and help your body heal itself, but currently there are no studies that confirm that polarity therapy actually achieves these goals.

How can I find a good polarity therapy practitioner?

To find a practitioner of polarity therapy, contact the American Polarity Therapy Association (see "Polarity Therapy" in Appendix B for more information). For $3.00, the association will send you an index of all their members, listed according to region.

Reflexology

Reflexology involves applying pressure to specific points on the soles of the feet, the palms of the hands, or the ears that are thought to correspond with various organs and other parts of the body. Reflexology theory maintains that the body is divided into ten zones, each running lengthwise from head to foot and down one arm through one of the ten fingers. Applying pressure on one part of the zone (the corresponding area of the foot, hand, or ear, for example) is believed to help relieve pain and encourage healing in another part of that zone.

The reflexologist will manipulate a specific area — most commonly on the bottom of the foot but sometimes on the palm of the hand or the ear — that corresponds to the diseased or painful area. He or she will use a map of the foot, hand, or ear that indicates the points that can stimulate healing in the heart, stomach, lung, pancreas, kidney, colon, eyes, ears, throat, and even the tonsils. For example, your reflexologist may press an area just outside the middle of the ball of your foot to stimulate your lungs. Reflexologists use special thumb, finger, and hand techniques, without the addition of oils or lotions, to stimulate your body parts. For most people, reflexology is a relaxing and pleasant experience.

What can reflexology do for me?

There are no studies that prove that reflexology is an effective treatment for arthritis. But, like most kinds of massage, reflexology may be helpful in reducing the stiffness seen in osteoarthritis and rheumatoid arthritis. It may also help increase circulation, which is helpful if you have Raynaud's phenomenon.

How can I find a good reflexologist?

Contact the Reflexology Association of America (See "Reflexology" in Appendix B) for referrals.

Touch therapy

In *touch therapy,* also known as therapeutic touch, energy is transmitted from the practitioner's hands to the patient's body to help speed the healing process and ease pain. Like certain Eastern philosophies, therapeutic touch is based on the belief that the body possesses an energy field and that the energy within this field must be ordered and balanced to maintain health. When the energy in this field becomes unbalanced, disease results.

Although the practitioner won't actually touch your body, he can discern where problems exist in your energy field by meditating while holding his hands over your body to feel the vibrations. The practitioner then channels energy into your body to help ease the pain and speed healing. One session usually takes about 30 minutes.

What can touch therapy do for me?

Some studies have found that therapeutic touch is effective, including one study performed on 25 patients with osteoarthritis. The participants in this study were divided into three groups: one received standard Western medical care, another received therapeutic touch, and a third received a simulated version of touch therapy. Those participants who actually received touch therapy experienced a significant decrease in pain along with an increase in mobility, while the other participants did not. However, other studies have shown that touch therapy has little or no effect. , In spite of this, therapeutic touch is taught at more than 80 different universities, is used by many nurses, and is the subject of a great deal of scientific research. If you're in pain, you may want to give it a try.

How can I find a good touch therapy practitioner?

To find a good touch therapy practitioner, contact the Nurse Healers — Professional Associates International, which is the official Therapeutic Touch organization. (See "Therapeutic Touch" in Appendix B for more information.)

Chapter 18

Ayurvedic Healing and Traditional Chinese Medicine

Two ancient healing arts were devised centuries before anyone knew of bacteria, EKGs, and blood counts. They come from India and China, where sophisticated societies flourished long before Western doctors donned their white coats.

The healing arts of India and China are based on philosophies foreign to Westerners; they seem somewhat odd and certainly unscientific. However, the two healing systems have many adherents, and many testify that they have been helped by either Ayurvedic healing or Traditional Chinese Medicine.

You should certainly have a medical doctor oversee your treatment, of course. But many have found that using Ayurvedic or traditional Chinese healing as adjuncts, under the direction of their physicians, has been quite helpful.

Ayurvedic Healing: "The Science of Life"

Some 5,000 years ago, healers and philosophers living on the subcontinent of India developed Ayurveda, also known as *science of life.* From there the *science of life* spread to China, Southeast Asia and other parts of the world, finally gaining some notice in the United States in the 1980s.

According to Ayurvedic thought, everyone contains greater or lesser amounts of the five elements that make up the entire universe: air, earth, water, fire, and *ether* (space). These five elements come together in the body to create the three *doshas* that can be defined as biologic humors or life forces: *vata, pitta,* and *kapha.* The three humors are everywhere inside the body, governing your physical and emotional health. They must always be in harmony; if the harmony is upset, you become ill. (But even if they remain in harmony, you may still become ill for other reasons, such as not maintaining good relationships, lack of attention to spiritual purpose, injury, hereditary factors, and so on.)

Just as everyone has unique fingerprints, everyone also has different mixes of *vata*, *pitta,* and *kapha.* The mix of the three determines your constitutional or *doshic* make-up, which in turn influences how your arthritis affects you and how it should be treated.

The goal of treatment

During your first visit to an Ayurvedic practitioner, she or he will ask a lengthy series of questions to help determine whether you are a *vata, pitta,* or *kapha*-type person. She or he will investigate your physical and emotional traits, habits, likes, and dislikes, as well as review your family history. After the question session comes the physical examination: your overall appearance, the way your pulse beats, the color of your tongue, and other physical attributes can provide *doshic* information.

If your Ayurvedic practitioner finds that any of the three *doshas* are out of balance, that is, if one has risen or fallen and the normal harmony is disturbed, she or he will try to adjust the balance and restore harmony.

Imbalances of the humors lead to disease, but it's not a simple matter of developing one disease if you're 10 percent low on *vata,* a different ailment if you're 15 percent "over" on *pitta,* and yet a third if you're 32 percent shy of the normal *kapha* level. Instead, the same disease presents itself differently, depending on the humor in which it strikes.

Although arthritis takes different forms with different symptoms, depending on which humor is out of balance, there is a common thread that ties the various forms of the disease together. It is believed that arthritis generally originates in the digestive system, caused by a cooling of the body's digestive fires, with a weakening of the colon and improper digestion. With the body unable to get all the nutrients it needs to keep itself clean, toxins build up and eventually harm the joints. That's why, regardless of the humor in which it strikes, the treatment for arthritis is designed to heat up the digestive fires and help the body burn off the toxins that are harming the joints.

Arthritis is essentially a problem of digestion and toxicity. Whether your disease is of the *vata*, *pitta*, or *kapha* type, your treatment includes proper diet, herbs, internal cleansing, exercise, massage, meditation, prayer, aromatherapy, water therapy, color therapy, yoga, and supplements — all designed to "reheat" the internal digestive fires and cleanse the body.

That's the basis of the general approach. But the specifics vary according to whether you have *vata-*, *pitta-,* or *kapha*-type arthritis.

While *doshic* imbalances are an important cause of arthritis, they are not the only reason we develop the ailment. For example, an injury or an errant immune system may be to blame.

Vata arthritis

Vata, the "air" humor, is a combination of air and ether. It tends to center in the colon, taking charge of our breathing, tissue, and muscle movement, heartbeat, and cell membranes. Associated with lightness and movement, *vata* encourages flexibility and creativity when it is properly balanced. When it is not, it triggers anxiety and fear. *Vata*-type people are more susceptible to arthritis, emphysema, flatulence, and other "air" diseases.

This *dosha* is dry, light, cold, active, and clear. When *vata* dominates, you typically find the following:

- ✔ Dryness in the body, in the hair, skin, colon, and so on. (Dryness in the colon can cause constipation.)
- ✔ A "light" body (small frame, underweight)
- ✔ Poor circulation, cold hands and feet
- ✔ Lots of physical movement and activity
- ✔ Clear thinking, quick understanding, and possibly clairvoyance
- ✔ Anxiety and insecurity

If arthritis manifests itself in the *vata* humor, it causes throbbing pain that hurts more when it's cold. The pain isn't constant; it waxes and wanes, it may move from one point to another. There's stiffness in the joints. If the problem isn't treated, the bones may become damaged. You may also suffer from gas, constipation, dry skin, fear, insomnia, and other problems.

The Ayurvedic doctor tries to reduce your *vata*, while strengthening your digestive fires. To do so, he may prescribe a three to five day detoxification diet. This may be followed by an anti-*vata* diet based on heavy, warm, moist foods that help build strength. He or she will ask you to eat many small meals with only a few foods per meal, go easy on the spices, and eat when calm and with friends.

Here are some of the specifics of the anti-*vata* diet and regimen:

- ✔ The diet consists of 50 percent whole grains, 20 percent protein (for example, eggs, fish, and tofu) and 30 percent fresh vegetables. You may exchange up to one-third of the vegetables for fresh fruit. Fish, chicken, and turkey help shrink *vata* down to proper levels, while beef, lamb, and pork do not.

- ✔ Helpful vegetables include cooked beets, carrots, parsley, potatoes, tomatoes, and onions, while vegetables that should be avoided include asparagus, broccoli, cabbage, cauliflower, eggplant, lettuce, and spinach.

- ✔ Mung beans are the only beans allowed because other kinds can aggravate *vata* ailments.

- ✔ Apples, cranberries, melons, and dried fruit should also be avoided.

- ✔ Couscous, oats, brown rice, and wheat are helpful, but barley, buckwheat, millet, rye, and dried grains are not.

- ✔ Choose warm foods and spices over cold foods. Warm dairy products are useful, as are small amounts of nuts or seeds, either raw or lightly roasted.

- ✔ Sweetness helps balance *vata*, so most sweeteners — except white sugar — are acceptable.

- ✔ Black pepper, cayenne, horseradish, garlic, nutmeg, ginger, basil, cinnamon, and other spices are good. Herbs such as licorice, ashwagandha, bala, brahmi, arjuna, guggul, rehmannia, zizphus, and sandalwood are also helpful.

- ✔ Plenty of fluid is essential, so sour fruit juice, milk, and herbal teas are encouraged. Before or during meals, small amounts of alcohol or herbal wines are helpful.

In addition to the dietary recommendations, you are advised to stay warm, remain calm, and establish and stick to a regular routine.

Pitta arthritis

Pitta is the "fire" humor, composed of fire and water. It plays a large role in body metabolism, governing digestion, absorption, and temperature, as well as the conversion of food into energy. When balanced, *pitta* encourages intelligence and understanding. When it is not, it can trigger anger and jealousy. *Pitta*-type people are more susceptible to inflammatory diseases.

This *dosha* is sharp, hot, liquid, sour, and oily. When *pitta* dominates, you typically find these traits:

- A sharp mind, good memory, sharp eyes, nose, and/or teeth
- A tendency to mature early
- Warm skin, early balding
- Strong body odor
- Oily skin, hair, and feces
- Ambition and an inclination to compare and compete

If arthritis manifests itself in the *pitta* humor, it may lead to burning pain made worse by heat. Other symptoms include swelling and inflammation, fever, a generalized feeling of heat, flushing of the skin, inappropriate sweating, irritability, and diarrhea.

When arthritis strikes in the *pitta* humor, the Ayurvedic doctor seeks to reduce your *pitta*, while strengthening your digestive fires. To do so, he or she may prescribe an anti-*pitta* diet based on heavy, cool, and slightly dry foods that are raw and plain. You will be asked to eat three full meals and avoid eating late at night.

Here are some of the details of the anti-*pitta* diet and lifestyle:

- The diet consists of 50 percent whole grains, 20 percent protein (for example, tofu, raw milk, the white meat of chicken or turkey, and cottage cheese), and 30 percent fresh vegetables. You may exchange up to a third of the vegetables for fresh fruit.
- Helpful vegetables include broccoli, brussel sprouts, cabbage, celery, potatoes, and okra. It's best to avoid certain vegetables, including onions, avocados, carrots, spinach, and watercress. You should eat vegetables steamed or raw.
- Beans are helpful but you should eat them plain, not spiced.
- Many fruits are helpful, including apples, cranberries, figs, oranges, and pears. You will have to avoid others, including papaya, bananas, peaches, cherries, and apricots.
- Spices tend to heat, which is the opposite of what you want when you have excess *pitta*. Therefore, only fennel, cilantro, mint, and a few other spices are allowed. Bala, brahmi, guduchi, manjistha, neem, and other herbs are helpful. Eat salt sparingly.
- Fluids are helpful in cooling *pitta's* heat. Vegetable and fruit juice, teas, and milk are generally recommended. You should avoid alcoholic beverages and spicy teas.
- Sweetness helps counteract excess *pitta*, so raw sugar and honey are useful. Avoid white sugar, old honey, and molasses.

> ✔ You can have most grains, with the exception of brown rice and buckwheat.
>
> ✔ You can have most dairy products, although you should avoid sour cream, ice cream, and a few others.
>
> ✔ Because *pitta* is oily, nuts and oils may be harmful, although you may eat small amounts of sunflower seeds. You should use oil sparingly, and then you should only use butter, corn oil, or coconut oil.

Do not become overheated. Avoid exposure to too much sun or steam. You can use ice packs to help cool the body. Exercise in the early morning or in the evening when the day's heat has faded.

Kapha arthritis

Kapha, composed of water and earth, makes up the bones, muscles, and other structural elements of the body, as well as the "glue" that keeps body cells intact. The "water" humor, *kapha* lubricates the joints and the rest of the body, and keeps the immune system strong. When in balance, *kapha* encourages love. When it's not in balance, *kapha* encourages greed and dangerous attachments. *Kapha*-type people are more susceptible to obesity, diabetes, and mucus-related ailments.

This *dosha* is slow, heavy, oily, and cool. When *kapha* dominates, you typically find:

> ✔ Slow metabolism
>
> ✔ "Weightiness" seen in the large frame, large muscles and/or excess body fat
>
> ✔ A strong appetite
>
> ✔ A strong memory, although *kapha* types are not mentally quick
>
> ✔ A tendency to move slowly, or not move at all
>
> ✔ A love of candy and other treats

If arthritis manifests itself in the *kapha* humor, it leads to a dull, achy pain that worsens with cold and dampness. Swollen joints are common, and there may also be mucus in the respiratory system and/or stool.

When arthritis strikes in the *kapha* humor, the Ayurvedic doctor seeks to reduce your *kapha* while strengthening your digestive fires. To do so, he or she may prescribe an anti-*kapha* diet based on warm, dry, light foods. He or she will prescribe three meals a day. The bulk of your food should be eaten between 10:00 in the morning and 6:00 in the evening, with lunch being the largest meal. He may also instruct you to fast at specific times.

Here are some of the guidelines for reducing excess *kapha*:

- The diet consists of 30-40 percent whole grains, 20 percent protein (for example, chicken, boiled or poached eggs, most beans, and limited goat milk), and 40-50 percent fresh vegetables. You may exchange up to a third of the vegetables for fresh fruit.

- Most of the protein should come from non-animal sources (such as beans). You should avoid beef, fish, lamb, and pork. You should only eat chicken and turkey in small amounts.

- Most vegetables are helpful, although you should eliminate "wet" foods such as tomatoes, cucumbers and sweet potatoes. You should eat all vegetables steamed and spiced.

- Kidney beans, adzuki beans, soybeans, lima beans, and other beans are helpful, as are lentils and split peas, because they are drying. You should avoid chickpeas, however.

- You should eliminate most fruits because they are watery. Some, such as apples, pears, and dried fruit, may be helpful.

- A few grains, such as barley and rye, are helpful. You should avoid most other grains.

- You need to keep consumption of dairy products to a minimum, except for goat's milk and a few others.

- While you may have pumpkin seeds and sunflower seeds, you should eliminate other seeds and nuts from your diet.

- Avoid oils as much as possible, using only small amounts of corn, soy, sunflower, and canola oil.

- Tea, spiced tea, and herbal tea are helpful. Drink only small amounts of water, and never cold or iced.

- Hot spices such as garlic, ginger, mustard, and cloves are helpful. Your Ayurvedic doctor may prescribe a variety of herbs, including bibitaki, guggul, myrrh, and motherwort. Avoid all sweeteners except honey.

In addition, stay active and exercise often.

The Limited Studies Are Encouraging

Although Ayurvedic healing has not yet been subjected to the rigorous scientific investigation Western medicine prefers, some studies on different elements of the healing art have been performed. For example, at least two studies indicate that a certain combination of Ayurvedic herbs helps reduce the pain of osteoarthritis, as well as the swelling, pain, and stiffness of rheumatoid arthritis. And certain Ayurvedic herbs may also help modify the course of rheumatoid arthritis by lowering the rheumatoid factor.

Traditional Chinese Medicine

Just like Ayurvedic healers, doctors of Chinese medicine strive to reestablish balance within the body. But instead of weighing one *dosha* against another, they seek to balance *yin* and *yang,* to make sure that the body's *chi*, moisture, and blood maintain a state of equilibrium and are flowing freely.

Yin and yang, the polar principles, are the feminine and masculine qualities that compose and unite everything and everyone. They are as Earth and Heaven, night and day, wet and dry, inner and outer; one cannot exist without the other, and neither must be allowed to dominate. When they are balanced, good health, productivity, good fortune, and other good things will follow.

According to Chinese medicine, the body is made up of three things:

- **Chi:** The force that animates us and allows to think, feel, and move.
- **Moisture:** Liquid that bathes, protects, and nourishes body tissue.
- **Blood:** More than the red fluid that flows in our arteries, in Traditional Chinese Medicine philosophy, it is the essential "stuff" from which the bones, skin, organs, muscles, and other parts of the body are made.

But Chinese medicine looks at more than the physical body. There's also spirit (*shen),* the spiritual manifestation that infuses everyone, and essence (*jing*), the regenerative and reproductive substance within us all. These five essential elements — chi, moisture, blood, spirit, and essence — must be nurtured and balanced if we are to remain in good health.

Determining the Type of Arthritis

Instead of classifying arthritis as osteoarthritis, rheumatoid arthritis, and so on, traditional Chinese medicine looks at this problem as one of imbalance. Every disease is the result of either the lack of or the congestion of chi, moisture, or blood. As a general rule, running short of one of these three essential elements can lead to recurrent illness, weakness, and poor digestion and/or blood flow. Congestion, on the other hand, may trigger aches and pains, swelling, distention of the belly, and/or irritability.

The balance and flow of chi, moisture, and blood can be affected by the following:

- **External pathogens:** Wind, cold, heat, damp, and dryness.
- **Mental pathogens:** Anger, anxiety, fear, and over-joy
- **Miscellaneous pathogens:** Poor diet, excess alcohol, lack of exercise, injury, and others.

To determine the type and cause of your internal imbalance, the traditional Chinese medicine doctor looks for patterns that tie your symptoms together. At the first examination, he carefully examines your complexion, body build, posture, tongue, skin, and fingernails, and checks your pulse in several places. To doctors of traditional Chinese medicine, the pulse reveals much more than how rapidly the heart is beating. For example, a slow pulse is related to diseases of cold, while a rapid pulse is related to diseases of heat. An irregular pulse suggests that the chi and blood have stagnated, while a superficial pulse is linked to problems caused by external pathogens.

The doctor also smells you, listens to the way you breathe and speak, and otherwise gathers physical clues. He may examine your urine and possibly your stool. The doctor will ask you numerous questions about your symptoms and bowel habits, what you eat, how much and how well you sleep, when and how you exercise, and so on. He will also explore your family history. All this is designed to discover the blockage, shortfall, or imbalance that has caused disharmony within your body.

The way your arthritis manifests in your body depends upon your particular "brand" of insufficiency or blockage. For example:

- *Migratory arthritis* seems to travel around the body, striking here and there. Patients with migratory arthritis are generally thinner, and their tongues may have a white coating. It usually begins when dampness, cold, and/or wind enter the body, interfering with the flow of blood and *chi*.

- *Painful arthritis* produces severe pain in one or more joints. Although it hurts, it usually does not produce inflammation. Painful arthritis strikes when the flow of *chi* and blood is slowed down by cold, and worsens with cold and inactivity.

- *Hot arthritis* makes the joints swell and become tender and painful. It is, in a sense, a secondary disease that strikes when excess heat is produced due to another ailment. With hot arthritis, the pulse is rapid and "slippery" (superficial), and there's a dry, yellow coating on the tongue.

Multifaceted Treatment

After the cause of the problem has been located, the doctor of Chinese Medicine may use a variety of techniques to restore balance, including:

- Diet
- Herbs
- Spices
- Acupuncture and acupressure (see Chapter 17)
- Tai chi chuan and other exercises

Pink is the color

A vital diagnostic tool to the doctor of traditional Chinese medicine, the tongue says a lot with its color and appearance. If you're in good health, the tongue is pink and has a clear coating. Here are some of the problems suggested by "off color" tongues:

✔ **Light coloration:** A lack of chi and blood.

✔ **Red:** Excess heat and accompanying diseases.

✔ **Purple-red:** Diseases of heat that have moved from the exterior to the interior of the body, or perhaps a lack of body fluid.

✔ **Purple or blue-purple:** Sluggish chi and blood.

Then there's the coating of the tongue:

✔ **White, greasy:** Problems related to cold, damp and/or phlegm.

✔ **Yellow, thick:** Chronic indigestion.

✔ **Yellow, greasy:** Problems related to internal heat and dampness or phlegm.

✔ **Gray-black:** Lack of body fluids caused by heat.

Prevention is a major part of Chinese medicine, so the doctor also spends time educating you in the ways of chi, yin, and yang, and other aspects of Chinese medicine philosophy.

If all goes well, your chi, moisture, blood, spirit, and essence will soon be in balance and flowing freely, allowing you to feel well again.

Chapter 19

Other Alternative Approaches

*W*e've looked into herbs, homeopathy, Oriental medicine, Ayurvedic healing, and "hands on" methods of healing such as, chiropractic, massage and trigger point therapy. But there are lots of other alternative methods that many people are currently using to ease the symptoms of arthritis. In this chapter, we'll take a look at these therapies, how they are performed, what they claim they can do for you, and where you can begin your search for a competent, qualified therapist. We make no endorsements or claims regarding these methods or any practitioners, individually or as a group. This list is simply for your information.

If you are lucky enough to find both a therapy that works and an excellent practitioner, it's still important that you continue to work with your physician and the other members of your health care team. Studies have shown that people with arthritis who completely ignore traditional medicine in favor of alternative methods find that their health deteriorates at an alarming rate. Remember: An alternative therapy should be used as a *complement* to traditional medicine, not as a substitute for it.

Aromatherapy

Aromatherapy uses a wide variety of fragrant substances called *essential oils* to treat physical and emotional ills. These oils are taken from the fruit, flowers, bark, or roots of plants, producing deliciously enticing smells that include the aromas of basil, bergamot, black pepper, camphor, cedar wood, chamomile, fennel, frankincense, hyssop, jasmine, juniper, lavender, patchouli, and rose. The unique aroma of each essential oil, when inhaled, is believed to trigger beneficial physiologic and emotional responses. Lavender, for example, is believed to be soothing and relaxing, which is why it's recommended for people who are stressed or anxious. Ginger, on the other hand, is thought to be energizing and warming and is sometimes used as a mild aphrodisiac.

How is it done?

Massage is perhaps the most effective delivery system for aromatherapy, using *carrier oils* that contain a small amount of one or more essential oils. Carrier oils are plain, unscented oils that do not irritate the skin (such as soy oil or corn oil) that make up the majority of the solution and applied to the skin, with only a drop or two of essential oil added for aromatic purposes. (With the exception of lavender oil, essential oils are never applied directly to the skin in their undiluted state because they are too strong and irritating.)

As pleasurable as an aromatherapy massage may be, it's certainly not the only way to enjoy the benefits of essential oils. Aromatic oils can also be dropped into a pot of boiling water and allowed to escape into the air in the form of steam, or the steam itself can be inhaled after the solution has cooled somewhat.

When inhaling steam, be sure to remove the pot from the stove and allow it to cool until the steam can be inhaled comfortably. Inhaling the steam from a boiling pot can cause burns!

What can it do for me?

Aromatherapy is an ancient healing art, dating back over 4,000 years to the ancient Egyptians who used fragrant oils to cure the ills of both mind and body. Plant oils were used throughout the Middle Ages to treat wounds and help heal disease. And modern proponents of aromatherapy insist that it can help treat acne, arthritis, bronchitis, poor circulation, skin problems, and many other conditions. Because it acts on the central nervous system, aromatherapy may also help to ease anxiety and depression, reduce stress, induce relaxation or sedation, ease pain, give you a lift, or even act as a mild stimulant.

The essential oils most often prescribed for arthritis pain include benzoin, birch, black pepper, chamomile, eucalyptus, ginger, and juniper. One study found that arthritis patients who used aromatherapy were able to reduce their intake of painkillers while maintaining thier current level of comfort.

How can I find a good aromatherapist?

Many people perform aromatherapy on their own, but it's a good idea to see a professional first to find out how to do it safely and effectively. You can find a certified aromatherapist by contacting one of the aromatherapy organizations listed in Appendix B.

Bee Venom Therapy

Believe it or not, this therapy uses the venom from bee stings to help alleviate your pain. Although the preferred method involves the sting of a live bee, the venom can also be administered via injection. But there are a few drawbacks to the injections — the FDA hasn't approved bee venom therapy as an antidote to pain, so you may have trouble finding a physician to treat you, and injections are believed to be less effective than the sting of a live bee.

How is it done?

The bee venom is administered either directly on or near the site of your pain, or on specific acupuncture points or trigger points. While the injections are pretty straightforward, applying the live sting of a bee is an interesting procedure. The bee, held in long tweezers, is placed on the designated spot and allowed to do its thing. (The area to be stung may be iced beforehand to dull the pain.) But this process may need to be repeated several times before you see any arthritis pain-relieving results. And, as you can imagine, it hurts.

What can it do for me?

Surprisingly, bee venom has powerful pain-relieving and anti-inflammatory effects. There are no human studies currently available to document its prowess, but it has been shown to help prevent induced arthritis in rats. Bee venom therapy is quite popular in Asia and Eastern Europe, and many people swear by its ability to ease the symptoms of their arthritis.

This treatment can be fatal if you develop an allergic reaction to the bee venom. Before beginning bee venom therapy, ask your doctor to test you for an allergy to bee stings. If you are allergic, do not use this treatment! And even if you aren't, it's imperative that you always have someone else present when you are stung, as well as an anaphylaxis emergency treatment kit (available by prescription only) in case you suddenly develop an allergic reaction.

How can I find a good bee venom therapy practitioner?

It's best to start with a physician who will give you bee venom injections, because the injections are less painful than the bee stings, and in case anything goes wrong, you'll already be in the presence of medical personnel. But bee venom isn't FDA-approved for this kind of therapy, so you may need to rely on word-of-mouth referrals or recommendations from a pain clinic to find a willing physician.

For live bee sting therapy, contact a beekeeper or other proponent of bee venom therapy. The American Apitherapy Society (see Appendix B) can provide you with information on this unusual therapy, how to administer it safely, and a list of members you can talk to who are familiar with the procedure.

Color Therapy

Long before the birth of Christ, the Egyptians were using colors to heal disease. They built rooms with specially designed windows that could break up the sun's rays into the colors of the rainbow, which were used in various medical and religious practices. Today, color is still being used for healing purposes. It's based on the belief that all objects radiate light of different wavelengths and applying the right kind of light to the body can restore balance and health.

How is it done?

The treatment begins with careful diagnosis and assessment of the color of the patient's eyes, skin, nails, urine, and stool. The color therapist also observes the way the patient speaks and acts and may use a special camera to study his or her aura. The patient and the color therapist will also discuss the patient's emotional and physical reactions to certain colors. After assembling this information, the color therapist diagnoses the condition and then attempts to heal the body by using various colors to counteract the problem.

Treatment consists of applying color to the body. One or more colors of light may be projected onto the affected areas, or the patient may be instructed to wear clothes or threads of a certain color or to eat and/or drink various foods or liquids of the desired color(s). Specific parts of the body might be touched with colored gems, and the patient may be asked to meditate on certain colors as a part of his or her therapy.

What can it do for me?

According to the theory of color therapy, color can affect the body in several ways. For example, it can be stimulating (red), cooling (blue), harmonizing and balancing (green), or cleansing and purifying (white).

Although there are no standard color therapies for arthritis, *blue* (soothing and cooling) is often used for rheumatism, *green* (calming to both mind and body) may be used to give hope and to increase energy, and *orange* (energy-releasing and restorative) may help treat gout, rheumatism, and diseases involving abnormal growths.

How can I find a good color therapist?

Unfortunately, you probably won't be able to find a color therapist by opening the Yellow Pages to *color,* because color therapy is usually performed in conjunction with other therapies, such as hypnosis or psychotherapy. See Appendix B, Resources under "Hypnotherapists," "Psychotherapy" or "The Mind/Body Connection" to find organizations that may be able to steer you to a color therapist.

DHEA (dehydroepiandrosterone)

This therapy is based on the belief that some kinds of arthritis may be related to a lack of a hormone called DHEA. Although DHEA is a male hormone (an androgen), it's manufactured in both male and female bodies. The body then uses DHEA to make several other hormones, including estrogen and testosterone. Levels of DHEA have been found to be low in some people with lupus, juvenile arthritis, and rheumatoid arthritis. So far, results have been positive when DHEA was given to women with mild to moderate forms of lupus. In one study of 191 women with lupus, 200 mg of DHEA per day helped ease fatigue, pain, and inflammation, allowing the women to cut back on their medication. Unfortunately, no scientific studies have yet shown the same positive results for rheumatoid or juvenile arthritis.

How does it work?

We don't know exactly how DHEA works against lupus. We do know, however, that the immune system "goes wild' in lupus, and that androgens tend to suppress immune function. Thus, DHEA may help combat some symptoms of lupus by keeping the immune system's "bad behavior" in check.

What can it do for me?

Besides helping to relieve symptoms of lupus, high levels of DHEA in the blood have been linked to a lower risk of heart disease, stroke, cancer, diabetes, Alzheimer's disease, and Parkinson's disease. Blood levels of DHEA decline rapidly after the age of 30, so keeping them high may help ward off degenerative diseases and age-related problems.

DHEA is a drug and may have side effects, therefore a physician should monitor its use. In some people, DHEA may increase the risk of cancer and heart disease. Do not take DHEA you're currently taking azathioprine (Imuran) or methotrexate, as the combination can cause liver damage.

How can I find DHEA?

Ask your doctor about DHEA. If he or she agrees that it may be worth a try, get a prescription. Some people need a dose of about 200 mg per day to see positive results, but it's best to start on a lower dosage and see what happens. DHEA is available in health food stores and other commercial enterprises, but steer clear of these varieties. Besides the fact that DHEA is a drug and a physician should always monitor its use, the quality and concentration of health food store varieties can vary quite a bit, so you can never quite be sure what you're getting.

You may see wild yam products in health food stores and catalogues that claim to be "natural," unprocessed sources of DHEA. But while they may be natural, your body cannot absorb DHEA until it has been chemically altered, so you may be wasting your money on them.

DMSD (dimethyl sulfoxide)

How can an industrial solvent that's used in paint thinner and antifreeze ease your arthritis pain? When used in its medical-grade form (as opposed to industrial-grade) it has anti-inflammatory and antioxidant properties, coupled with a remarkable ability to transport substances through cell membranes. Some studies have shown that DMSO can ease muscle and joint pain, relax constricted blood vessels seen in Raynaud's phenomenon, heal the skin ulcers seen in scleroderma, and soften scleroderma's hardened collagen deposits.

How is it used?

DMSO, a clear liquid, can be applied externally, swallowed, or injected into veins or muscles. It can be rubbed onto the skin to ease inflammation of the joints and soft tissues. It can help other drugs cross cell membranes and can even soften collagen. But whether taken internally or externally, DMSO has a couple of unpleasant (although harmless) side effects: Those who take it smell like a combination of oysters and garlic, and it leaves a bad taste in the mouth.

What can it do for me?

DMSO was considered a revolutionary new treatment for arthritis when it was introduced back in the 1960s. But in the mid-1960s, animal studies involving very high doses of DMSO showed it also caused damage to the lens of the eye (although no studies have shown eye problems in humans). DMSO quickly fell out of favor, and today many American physicians don't use it except to treat a bladder ailment known as interstitial cystitis. DMSO is still being used regularly to treat osteoarthritis and rheumatoid arthritis in Russia and some other countries, however.

How can I find DMSO?

You and your physician need to have an in-depth discussion about the pros and cons of DMSO usage before you decide whether you want to try it. If you do decide to try it, you should do so only under medical supervision. Although it's possible to purchase DMSO over the counter, chances are it is not in a purified form; thus, it may be too strong and/or detrimental to your health. There is a DMSO treatment program available through Oregon Health Sciences University where you can contact Dr. Stanley Jacob (the doctor who brought DMSO to the public's attention in the 1960s) for more information. (See Appendix B, Resources under "DMSO/MSM.")

MSM (methylsulfonylmethane)

When DMSO is broken down within the body, about 15 percent of it becomes MSM, which holds on to many of the same benefits of DMSO but has fewer detriments. For example, it doesn't produce the oyster/garlic smell on the breath, doesn't appear to damage the body in any way and doesn't require a prescription. Yet it does seem to help fight inflammation, and may help alleviate some of the symptoms of RA.

How is MSM used to treat arthritis?

MSM is available in capsule or lotion form. The standard dose for capsules is 1,000 mg twice a day, but a starting dose of 500 mg twice a day is a better idea, while you watch for side effects. If all goes well, gradually increase the amount until you reach the standard dose. Consult your physician before taking MSM, however, and make sure that she or he monitors your health with regular blood tests to assess liver and kidney function. Do not stop taking your arthritis medication(s) unless advised to do so by your physician.

MSM and DMSO may produce blood-thinning effects and if used in conjunction with blood-thinners such as heparin, aspirin, or certain herbs, can cause excessive bleeding or prolonged clotting time. Consult your physician about adverse interactions before taking either MSM or DMSO.

What can it do for me?

When James Coburn won the Academy Award for Best Supporting Actor in 1999, he gave the marketing campaign for MSM a real shot in the arm by claiming that MSM had made it possible for him to fight the pain and disability of rheumatoid arthritis and continue working. Since then, MSM has been touted as a pain-relieving and inflammation-fighting treatment for osteoarthritis, rheumatoid arthritis, gout, and fibromyalgia. Its advertisers also claim that it can neutralize an acid stomach, fight allergies, and ease constipation, among other things. The problem is, there is no real scientific proof of any of this. A great deal more research is needed before it can be said that it's safe. One thing we do know is that any benefits conferred by MSM tend to disappear if the supplement is no longer taken.

How can I find MSM?

The same physician who uncovered new and exciting uses for DMSO also developed MSM. You can contact Dr. Stanley Jacob through Oregon Health Sciences University for more information. (See Appendix B, Resources under "DMSO/MSM.")

Folk Medicine

Folk medicine is "homemade" therapy — the kind your great-grandma probably practiced 100 years ago to treat a stuffy nose, heart palpitations, constipation, and everything in between. It's a giant, catchall category made up of remedies both ancient and modern that borrows from the religious beliefs and practical experiences of people throughout the world. Folk medicine may call for herbs, food, drink, prayer, and/or rituals, and (like most things that have lasted for centuries) it does have some merit. American Indians, for example, used to chew willow bark to relieve toothaches: Today we know that willow bark contains a form of aspirin. And the foxglove plant, a centuries-old folk remedy for heart problems, is the basis for the modern heart medication *digitalis*.

How is folk medicine used to treat arthritis?

There are many folk medicine treatments for arthritis, including drinking apple cider vinegar, sipping raw potato juice, downing a combination of blackstrap molasses and water, rubbing raw ginger or garlic on painful joints, or applying poultices to the affected area made of potatoes, mustard, and castor oil.

What can it do for me?

According to folk wisdom, drinking the potions previously listed can increase overall health and vitality while easing joint pain. Eating raw ginger or garlic may help "warm" the joints and reduce stiffness by increasing circulation, and poultices are supposed to "draw out the pain" from aching joints.

How can I find a good folk medicine practitioner?

Your best bet is consulting with a naturopathic physician. Naturopaths (N.D.s) are not licensed to prescribe drugs or perform major surgery like medical doctors, but they do go through a rigorous four-year program that includes training in herbal medicine, homeopathy, nutrition, hydrotherapy, and other natural methods of treating illness. Naturopaths are more likely than medical doctors to use folk remedies, and they also tend to make practical use of the most recent research in nutrition, botanicals, homeopathy, and other natural treatments. You can find a naturopathic physician by contacting one of the organizations listed under "Naturopathic Medicine" in Appendix B, Resources.

Hydrotherapy

Hydrotherapy is an ancient treatment using water (both hot and cold), steam, and ice to stimulate and soothe the body, thus rearranging its energies and encouraging healing.

How is it done?

Water is applied to the entire body or just to specific areas in the form of liquid, steam, or ice. It may be delivered via showers, baths, sitz baths, warm and cool compresses, wet sheet wraps, hot blankets, saunas, and other techniques. Hydrotherapy can also be performed internally by drinking water and/or taking colonics (enemas that flush out the colon).

What can it do for me?

Hydrotherapy is an age-old therapy for arthritis. The Romans were famous for their public baths, where people "took the waters" to ease the pain of arthritic joints. A modern hydrotherapist may recommend a variety of treatments, including colonics to rid the body of toxins, drinking plenty of distilled water to flush toxins away, taking short cold baths or showers to increase circulation, using warm baths, saunas, or steam rooms to increase circulation and sweat out toxins, and applying cold compresses to ease joint pain.

Although bathing in mineral waters (and sometimes drinking them) has long been touted as a health aid, there is little evidence to suggest that bathing in plain old warm water doesn't do just as well!

How can I find a good hydrotherapist?

To find a specialist in hydrotherapy, contact one of the organizations listed under "Massage Therapists" or "Naturopathic Medicine" in Appendix B, Resources. Be sure to look for one experienced in treating arthritis, as some forms of hydrotherapy may be detrimental to your condition (for example, cold water therapy for Raynaud's phenomenon).

Is Alternative Medicine for You?

Deciding whether or not to experiment with alternative therapies is a very individual matter and will depend on many things: How dissatisfied you are with traditional Western therapies, how adventurous you are, how willing you are to try unproven or controversial methods, what your inner voice tells you, and how your body responds.

If you should opt for alternative treatments, always remember that many of them (if any) are *not* supported by reams of scientific studies, so you'll be taking a chance. Always research any therapy you'd like to try (in advance), find yourself the best-qualified and most highly recommended practitioner, consult with your physician before and during treatment, and make sure that your physician monitors your progress. But perhaps the most important thing you can do is to listen to your body. Are you feeling better? Does this approach seem to be working? Sometimes even the most scientifically sound method won't help you, while something strange and virtually inexplicable will. Your body possesses its own brand of wisdom — let it speak to you.

Part V
The Part of Tens

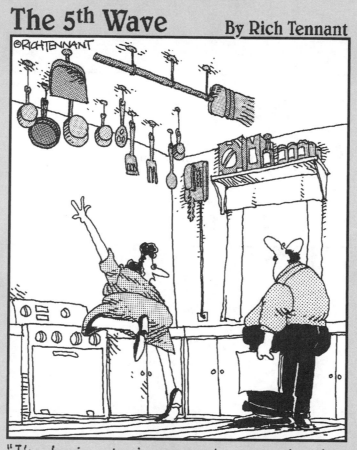

The 5th Wave   By Rich Tennant

"I'm trying to incorporate more stretching and ROM exercises into my daily routine."

In this part . . .

This part of the book is a kind of "distilled" way of presenting some key information on managing your arthritis. We include ten arthritis myths, ten tips for management and prevention of arthritis, ten super foods that can help you fight arthritis, and ten crackerjack new treatments that you might not have heard about yet.

Chapter 20

Ten Myths about Arthritis

*A*rthritis has been plaguing mankind for centuries, so people have had plenty of time to figure out ways to define it, explain it, and attempt to make it disappear. But some of these theories have turned out to be pure bunk — ill-founded beliefs that go head-to-head with proven facts. Still, some of these myths manage to hang on stubbornly, and you'll hear them repeated by friends, family members, and even health care givers as if they had some sort of scientific basis. But once you've read through this list, *you* will know better.

Only Old Folks Get Arthritis

Although we tend to think of arthritis as the joint stiffness, aches, and pains that Grandma suffers from, the fact is that arthritis affects people in all age groups, and a full two-thirds of them are under the age of 65. Arthritis is the nation's leading cause of disability among those over the age of 15. The 355 million people worldwide who are affected by arthritis are *not* just senior citizens, as you can see by this breakdown of the rest of the population:

Children: The Arthritis Foundation estimates that arthritis affects, some 285,000 children, who may develop juvenile rheumatoid arthritis, ankylosing spondylitis, juvenile forms of lupus, and other kinds of arthritis. Children between the ages of 5 and 15 are one of the two groups most likely to suffer from polymyositis.

Women in the childbearing years: Close to 90 percent of all cases of lupus are developed by women between the ages of 15 and 40. Women in this age category are also seven times more likely than men to develop fibromyalgia.

Men age 20-40: Ankylosing spondylitis, a disease affecting some 300 thousand Americans, has targeted young to middle-aged men as its favorite group. Young men are also more likely to develop activity-related arthritis, such as the Lyme disease often contracted by hikers who have sustained bites from infected ticks, or gonoccoccal arthritis, and/or Reiter's syndrome, which can result from unprotected sex.

Women and men age 30-60: Polymyositis, which causes inflammation and severe weakness of the muscles, favors those in this age group, attacking women twice as often as men. These are also the years that osteoarthritis, due to old sports injuries or other joint abuse, is likely to surface. Rheumatoid arthritis is also liable to strike in middle age.

Arthritis Is Just a Minor Problem

If only it were so! The truth, however, is that arthritis is a major-league problem that exceeds or equals virtually any other health problem in the nation. It affects one out of six Americans (about 43 million people) and is the number one cause of disability in the United States. And the ranks of arthritis sufferers are growing — by 2020, experts estimate that one out of five Americans will be affected, or almost 60 million people.

More than 7 million Americans must limit their daily living activities (such as walking, cooking, housework, and driving) due to arthritis, and 43 to 85 percent of RA victims find themselves permanently unable to work eight to eleven years after diagnosis. The cost to our nation in medical visits, disability, and days lost from work due to arthritis has been estimated at $65 billion a year, an amount equal to a mid-level recession.

While osteoarthritis may not be a life-threatening disease, consisting mostly of "aches and pains," many kinds of arthritis can destroy joint tissue, affect the internal organs, severely limit physical and financial independence, and even reduce life expectancy. Because this is such a serious disease, early diagnosis and proper treatment are essential.

Arthritis Only Affects the Joints

Osteoarthritis, the most common form of arthritis, is primarily a joint disease. But other forms of arthritis can attack parts of the body that have nothing to do with the joints. Rheumatoid arthritis can damage the lungs, heart, or eyes. JRA triggers eye inflammation, swollen lymph nodes, and inflammation of the linings of the lungs and heart. And psoriatic arthritis is usually accompanied by a scaly skin condition. Although the symptoms of arthritis can vary widely, the one thing all of them have in common is pain in and around the joints.

Exercise Worsens Arthritis

In the old days, when Grandpa's "rheumatism" acted up or Grandma suffered from arthritis aches and pains, they tended to retire to the rocking chair and just wait it out. Today we know that exercise is one of the best medicines for relieving joint pain and stiffness, increasing range of motion and mobility, and keeping arthritis pain at bay. This is especially true for osteoarthritis, which can leave the cartilage thin, dry, and degenerated. When you exercise, joint fluid replete with nutrients and life-giving water is forced into and out of the cartilage, bringing in nourishment and taking away wastes. This keeps the cartilage moist and well fed, while the joint supporting structures are simultaneously strengthened and stretched. Healthy joints absolutely depend on exercise, but that doesn't mean they have to bear weight at the same time. If you're experiencing a flare, you can exercise in the water without putting pressure on your joints.

Gout Means You Eat Too Much Meat

Gout used to be referred to as the "rich man's disease" because it occurred most often in wealthy men who could afford to eat rich foods and expensive meats (and who, accordingly, often became overweight in the process). But today we know that gout is a metabolic disorder causing a build-up of uric acid in the blood, and that uric acid crystals tend to settle in the big toe, with excruciating results. Although a diet high in purines (found in meats and certain seafoods such as anchovies, herring, mackerel, sardines, and scallops) increases the uric acid level and can make gout worse, diet alone is not the cause.

Wearing Copper Bracelets Cures Arthritis Pain

Here's a good ol' myth that's been around for ages and will probably hang in for the long haul because it's cheap, it can't hurt you, and some people swear it works. All you have to do is wear a copper bracelet, ring, or disc (that can be glued to the back of your watch), and your body will absorb some of that copper straight through the skin, which is supposed to relieve your pain.

In reality, it's doubtful that your skin is able to absorb copper just from contact with a copper bracelet or ring — and even it does, you probably don't need the extra copper. If you do happen to be copper deficient, taking a multimineral containing copper is a much more direct and efficient way to handle the problem.

Yet a placebo-controlled study involving 300 people, half of whom wore copper bracelets and half of whom wore bracelets that only looked like copper found that a significant number of those who wore the real thing got some pain relief. So who can say for sure?

Although science can't confirm the pain relieving effects of copper bracelets, it appears to be harmless and might be worth a try. But make sure the copper bracelet or ring you buy hasn't been lacquered, for the lacquer will form a barrier between your skin and the metal. (If your copper jewelry stays bright and shiny, rather than turning a dark, murky brown like an old penny, it's been lacquered.)

Eating Alfalfa Reduces Arthritis Symptoms

Alfalfa, which most people think of as the stuff cattle munch on, is an excellent overall health booster. It's rich in calcium, beta-carotene, magnesium, and potassium; it's a natural diuretic and laxative, as well as an appetite stimulant. In folk medicine, eating alfalfa has long been recommended for reducing the swelling and inflammation of arthritis.

While consuming lots of alfalfa won't necessarily relieve your arthritis symptoms, it may actually have some dangerous side effects. Because it's a rich source of Vitamin K, which helps promote blood clotting, alfalfa can interfere with your normal clotting mechanism, as well as with normal blood cell production. And in animal experiments, alfalfa has been shown to aggravate the symptoms of lupus, so those who have lupus, rheumatoid arthritis, or other autoimmune diseases should stay away from it.

Eggplant and Other "Nightshade" Vegetables Cause Arthritis

"Nightshade" vegetables come from the *Solanum* plant genus, made up of more than 1,700 trees, herbs and shrubs. The genus includes the plants that produce potatoes, eggplant, tomatoes, and bell peppers. Back in the 1960s, a horticulturist from Rutgers University noticed that when he ate these vegetables his joints ached, but when he removed them from his diet, he felt better.

The myth that arthritis can be cured by eliminating nightshades from the diet spread far and wide, and you may still get wind of it today. But throughout the 40-year life of this theory, not a shred of scientific proof has ever been produced. In fact, you might do yourself a disservice if you cut these nutritious foods out of your diet, because you'll deprive yourself of some much-needed vitamins, minerals, and fiber.

Everyone Gets Arthritis Eventually

Experts estimate that arthritis affects about 2 percent of those aged 45 and younger, 25 to 30 percent of those 46 to 65, and anywhere from 65 to 85 percent of those 66 and older. But even among the oldest group, 15 to 35 percent may remain untouched by the disease. Whether or not you develop arthritis will depend a lot upon your genetic makeup and how you've treated your joints over the years. But as we gain greater knowledge of this disease and learn better methods of prevention, we look forward to increasing the number of people who manage to stay "arthritis-free" throughout their lives.

You Can't Treat Arthritis Successfully

Although most forms of arthritis cannot be eradicated, major scientific advances in recent years have made treatment of the disease much more effective, thus correcting deformities, restoring function, and easing pain as never before. Gout, for example, was once a debilitating and extremely painful form of arthritis that one simply had to endure. But today's medications can keep it almost completely under control. Surgery to replace worn, damaged, or painful joints has given thousands of people new leases on life, restoring movement and function that could only be dreamed about in the past. Newer, more effective medications can do much to relieve pain, inflammation, and other troubling symptoms in various kinds of arthritis, ranging from RA to osteoarthritis to Lyme disease. And exciting new developments in genetics are being revealed regularly that increase our understanding of the origins of this disease, how best to treat it, and how to prevent its onset.

Chapter 21

Ten Ways to Prevent and Manage Arthritis

In This Chapter

▶ A wrap-up of some of the most important topics in this book

▶ How to take care of your arthritic joints today

▶ How to prevent onset or progression of arthritis tomorrow

*I*ncluded in this book are hundreds of ways to manage your arthritis, from bee venom thereapy to bed rest, from NSAIDs to nightshades, from TENS to total joint replacement surgery. But the most important points for you to remember can be distilled into what we call the Ten Commandments of Arthritis Management.

Signs? Symptoms? See Your Doctor

The sooner you begin treatment, the greater your chances of preventing or at least slowing the damage to your joints. Medical science is making great strides in arthritis treatment, but you won't be able to take advantage of these new discoveries until you're under a doctor's care. Some experts have estimated that the greatest amount of joint damage occurs during the first two years after onset of the disease. Don't wait — help is available if you ask for it.

See your doctor if you have any of these symptoms in a joint or its surrounding tissues for more than two weeks:

- ✔ Pain
- ✔ Stiffness
- ✔ Swelling
- ✔ Trouble bending and/or flexing a joint

Exercising Regularly for Strength and Flexibility

We just can't stress this enough! Regular physical activity strengthens joint support structures, helping them take some of the pressure off the joint itself, while nourishing and moisturizing the cartilage. Aerobic activity can tone you all over, strengthen your heart, increase bone density, and help you keep your weight under control (very important, especially for those with arthritis of the knee). Flexibility (stretching) exercises increase and maintain your range of motion, loosen up your muscles, and make your tendons and ligaments more resilient. At the same time, these exercises help release tension and promote relaxation. All of this translates into less pain and stiffness, greater ease of movement, and an improved mental attitude. In addition, exercise can increase your physical abilities, help prevent joint deformities, boost your immune system, improve your balance, and help you maintain your independence. We wish that we could bottle it!

Adopting Healthy Eating Habits

Eating a healthful, balanced diet is important for everybody, but especially if your body is stressed by an ongoing condition. Arthritis sufferers may need to be especially careful about what they eat because some foods can actually make their conditions worse while other foods can help relieve some of their symptoms.

In general, you should try to do the following:

- Eat a wide variety of foods, focusing on whole grains, fresh fruits, and fresh vegetables, with smaller amounts of meat, fish, poultry, (four to six ounces per day maximum) and dairy products.
- Limit your intake of cholesterol, fat, sugar, and salt (sodium)
- Take it easy on the alcohol.
- Use olive oil, canola oil, flaxseed oil and others high in the "good" fatty acid (linoleic acid), which can help lessen inflammation.
- Watch your intake of foods that contain the "bad" fatty acid (arachidonic acid) such as meat, poultry, egg yolks, and full-fat dairy products.
- Eat fish that contain omega-3 fatty acids (mackerel, herring, salmon, and so on) a couple of times weekly.

Managing Your Weight: Joint Infrastructure

Carrying too much body weight is a major contributor to osteoarthritis of the weight-bearing joints, especially the knee. Lessening the "load" exerted by excess weight automatically eases osteoarthritis pain and movement limitation in these important joints.

The best way to lose weight is to follow the Food Pyramid guidelines for a good diet and increase your exercise. In general, try to limit foods that are calorically dense (fats and sweets) and make every bite count. Eat highly nutritious foods that are worth their calories (for example one-half cup yogurt instead of one-half cup ice cream; one tablespoon peanut butter instead of one tablespoon butter). Don't starve, fast, skip meals, or try to cut back too drastically. These methods are almost guaranteed to fail. Just cut back on sweets, fats, and portion sizes a little, while increasing your exercise a little. If you don't see results on the scale and/or around your waistline in two weeks, cut back a little more and step up the exercising. Once you begin to lose pounds, just keep on doing what you're doing. You're on the right track!

Using Joint Protection Techniques

The way you use (or abuse) your joints day in and day out can greatly help or hinder joint health. Remember (and use) these joint protection techniques recommended by the Arthritis Foundation:

- Respect pain.
- Avoid joint stressing postures or positions.
- Avoid staying in one position for a long time.
- Use the strongest and largest joints and muscles for the job.
- Avoid sustained joint activities.
- Maintain muscle strength and joint range of motion.
- Use assistive devices or splints, if necessary.

Taking Medication When Indicated

The right medication can make a world of difference to the quality of your life and, in some cases, the rate at which your arthritis progresses. Pain relievers (analgesics and/or NSAIDs) can help control the aches and pains that make it so difficult for you to get through the day and enjoy life. Other drugs, such as DMARDs (disease modifying antirheumatic drugs) reduce inflammation and help prevent or slow joint damage and destruction.

Your physician will tell you if medication is appropriate for your condition and if it can help ward off complications down the road. If medication is indicated, take it religiously, following your doctor's instructions to letter. Good compliance can pay big dividends, today and in the future.

Consider Taking Supplements

Together, glucosamine and chondroitin sulfate increase production of collagen, the "framework" of cartilage; slow certain enzymes that prematurely destroy cartilage; block enzymes that interfere with the transfer of nutrients to the cartilage; and increase the production of proteoglycans, the molecules that help keep cartilage "wet" and healthy.

Among some of the other supplements that may help fight arthritis are the following:

- **Fish oil (containing omega-3 fatty acids):** To help ease symptoms of rheumatoid arthritis, prevent the spasms seen in Raynaud's syndrome and relieve some symptoms of lupus.
- **Evening primrose, borage, or black current oils (containing gamma-linolenic acid):** To reduce the pain and inflammation seen in rheumatoid arthritis, and ease the pain of scleroderma, while improving the skin texture.
- **Boron:** To reduce symptoms of osteoarthritis.
- **Vitamin B$_6$:** To relieve the pain and stiffness of carpal tunnel syndrome.
- **Niacin:** To reduce the frequency and duration of attacks of Raynaud's syndrome.
- **Zinc:** To reduce symptoms of rheumatoid arthritis and ease the joint pain of psoriatic arthritis.

And many, many more. Once your doctor has okayed your use of supplements, feel free to experiment, but stay with recommended dosages and discontinue their use if you become aware of any undesirable side effects.

Balancing Rest and Activity

This is a very important part of any arthritis management program — and it can be more difficult than you think. Too much rest is bad for your body. You need activity (exercise) to keep your cardiovascular system in shape, your weight down, your joint supporting structures strong, your cartilage "lubed," and to maintain or increase your range of motion. But too much exercise can aggravate your arthritis symptoms and cause injury. Only you will be able to determine how much of each is too much. One thing, however, is certain: If you're having a flare, you'll need to cut back on your activity. But try to get back in the exercise game as soon as possible to build and maintain your fitness.

Feeling Pain? Stop!

"Feel the burn" was a popular saying in fitness classes in the 1980s, but the burn they were referring to wasn't supposed to be in your joints! If you feel joint pain, it's time to rest, change activities, and maybe even call it a day. The last thing you want is to damage your joints even more.

Consider Surgery, If Applicable

Recent years have seen dramatic improvements in joint surgery. Today joints can be realigned, surgically stabilized, or even completely rebuilt. Diseased joint linings can be removed and fresh, new cartilage cells can be implanted. Arthroscopic techniques have turned what used to be major surgery into a nearly non-invasive procedure. And many, many people have experienced significant decreases in pain accompanied by remarkable increases in function.

If you have exhausted every possible means of managing your arthritis, if pain and poor joint function are severely compromising the quality of your life, and if your kind of arthritis responds well to surgery, you may want to consider it seriously. Of course, the decision to have surgery should not be made lightly, and the pros and cons must be carefully weighed. If you opt for surgery, you'll want to get the most qualified, highly-recommended surgeon you can find. Think about it, but make sure it's truly a last resort.

Chapter 22

Ten Super Foods to Fight Arthritis

- -

In This Chapter

▶ How fish can help relieve some arthritis symptoms

▶ How carrots bring all-over benefits that aren't just confined to your eyes

▶ The link between spinach and joint pain

▶ How an apple a day can do more than simply keep the doctor away

- -

*A*lthough diet alone cannot cure arthritis, certain nutrients have been linked to healthy joints. Low levels of these nutrients have been associated with joint pain, stiffness, and other problems, and several studies have shown that replacing what's missing can help relieve symptoms.

Here are ten super foods that can help fight the battle against arthritis by providing some of the nutrients that are known to be useful. While none of these foods actually gets rid of your arthritis, the nutrients they contain may be able to help you feel better.

Fish

Studies have shown that the omega-3 fatty acids found in certain fish can help reduce the pain of osteoarthritis, as well as the joint stiffness and tenderness seen in rheumatoid arthritis. The omega-3 fatty acids are believed to help fight arthritis by "dampening" the inflammation response, thus reducing joint pain and tenderness. In one study, women with rheumatoid arthritis were compared to women of the same age who did not have the disease. The researchers found that women who ate more than one serving of grilled or baked fish (other than tuna) per week had less risk of developing rheumatoid arthritis than those who did not.

The Arthritis Foundation agrees that omega-3s can help in the battle against arthritis, especially rheumatoid arthritis, and to some extent Raynaud's syndrome and lupus. Good fish sources of omega-3 fatty acids include mackerel (Atlantic, Pacific, and Spanish), herring (Atlantic and Pacific), salmon (king, Chinook, and pink) and roe. Some "non-fish" foods also contain omega-3 fatty acids, such as green soybeans, black walnuts, and flaxseed oil.

> ## Eskimos and omega-3s
>
> Here's a "fish story" for you that isn't a tall tale! In the 1970's, researchers began to study the diets of Eskimos, who had very little coronary heart disease despite eating tons (well, all right, pounds) of very fatty fish on a regular basis. Not only that, they ate relatively little fiber, fresh fruits, and vegetables. According to the best medical wisdom, they should have been dropping from heart attacks right and left. But they weren't.
>
> Over time, the researchers realized that the omega-3 fatty acids found in fish could help protect the heart. As research continued, they also discovered that the omega-3s could help maintain blood pressure at proper levels, combat ulcerative colitis, keep diabetes under control, and help relieve arthritis pain and stiffness.

Mackerel may be troublesome for those with gout, and too much fish oil can hamper the ability of the blood to clot.

Apples

Everybody knows that "an apple a day keeps the doctor away," but did you know that apples can also help fight arthritis?

Apples contain a good amount of a largely overlooked mineral called boron, an important factor in bone and joint health. Folks usually associate calcium with bones. Many women take calcium supplements specifically to keep their bones strong and stave off osteoporosis. But calcium can't do it alone; it needs the help of several other vitamins and minerals, including boron.

There is no direct link between boron and arthritis. That is, we can't show that if you run short of boron you will absolutely get arthritis, or that giving boron to those with the disease will solve their problems. But we do know that people with osteoarthritis tend to have less boron in their bones and synovial fluid than do non-arthritics. We also know that there is more osteoarthritis seen in populations with diets containing less than 1 mg of boron per day than in populations with daily diets containing 3 to 10 mg of boron.

Apples are a good — and tasty — source of boron. You'll also find this mineral in broccoli and other leafy vegetables, pears, peaches, grapes, nuts, and legumes.

Spinach and Other Green Leafy Vegetables

Remember when Popeye would squeeze open a can of spinach, gulp it down, and his muscles would double, triple, or maybe even quadruple in size? Suddenly, it was no sweat for him to defeat his enemies with a single punch.

Unfortunately, eating spinach won't dispatch arthritis as quickly as Popeye does Brutus, but the vitamin E found in this vegetable can help relieve some of the symptoms of the following different types of arthritis:

- **Rheumatoid arthritis:** At least one study has shown that vitamin E can be as effective as an NSAID in reducing the pain of rheumatoid arthritis. Vitamin E may also be helpful in relieving pain in rheumatoid patients who are already being treated with anti-rheumatoid drugs.

- **Osteoarthritis:** Vitamin E seems to inhibit the prostaglandins that help "stir up" inflammation. By helping to control inflammation, the vitamin may behave like the NSAIDs prescribed to relieve arthritis pain. In two studies, vitamin E was found to be more effective than a placebo in relieving osteoarthritis pain.

- **Fibromyalgia:** Way back in 1949, 300 middle-aged fibromyalgia patients were given mixed tocopherols (a form of vitamin E). Symptoms in the majority of these patients improved.

- **Lupus:** In several small studies, lupus lesions improved when patients were given up to 1,600 IU of vitamin E daily. And in one study conducted during the summer (when the lesions may get worse), the lesions seemed to remain stable.

Spinach has other benefits. It contains alpha linolenic acid, an omega-3 fatty acid that helps combat inflammation. It also has excellent amounts of folic acid, which is depleted in many arthritis patients who take large amounts of aspirin. And its vitamin E may help relieve some arthritis aches and pains.

Carrots

Carrots originally came from Afghanistan, where they were scrawny and came in a variety of colors (including black!). They contain excellent amounts of beta carotene, the "plant form" of vitamin A that is converted into vitamin A once it's inside the body.

Some case histories suggest that beta carotene can help reduce lupus-induced sensitivity to the sun. Carrots can also indirectly combat problems associated with taking NSAIDS. Some people take antacids to counteract the stomach distress caused by NSAIDs, but antacids can interfere with your body's ability to absorb the mineral phosphorus. You need phosphorus to keep your bones strong, build cells walls, convert carbohydrates, protein, and fat into energy, and otherwise keep the body running smoothly. Cooked carrots provide good amounts of phosphorus and can help you rebuild your stores of the mineral.

Cantaloupe

The cantaloupe, named for its hometown of Cantalupa, Italy, is an excellent source of vitamin C and beta carotene, the "plant form" of vitamin A. One-half of a medium sized cantaloupe contains over 180 percent of the RDA for vitamin C, and about 85 percent of the RDA for beta carotene (vitamin A). All that beta carotene can help reduce lupus-related sun sensitivity, while vitamin C may help combat arthritis-related inflammation.

Grapefruit and Other Citrus Fruits

Quercetin, hesperidin, rutin: These are just three of the many bioflavonoids found in the skin, peel, and outer layers of citrus fruits and leafy vegetables, as well as in wine, coffee, and tea.

Among other things, the bioflavonoids help increase capillary strength and permeability, fight inflammation, inhibit viruses, and strengthen the collagen that's so important to joint health.

Garlic

Almost 150 years ago, Louis Pasteur noted that garlic killed some of the bacteria in his laboratory petri dishes. Since then we've learned a great deal more about this aromatic food, including one piece of "accidental" information: Garlic can help relieve joint pain. Doctors noticed this when they were using it to treat heart disease. Some of their patients who also suffered from arthritis reported that their joint pain had subsided since they had been taking the garlic. Because garlic has not yet been studied in large-scale arthritis trials, exactly why and how well it works remains a mystery.

Papaya

Many people with arthritis and arthritis-related conditions take large amounts of aspirin to help relieve their pain and reduce swelling. Aspirin is an effective medicine, but it has several side effects. One of these is to lower the body's stores of vitamin C, a vitally important vitamin and antioxidant. Making sure you have plenty of C is important, because the vitamin has been linked to a slower rate of joint deterioration due to osteoarthritis. In one ten-year study, people with osteoarthritis of the knee who had been taking the most vitamin C showed the least disease progression. People looking for a tasty way to replenish their vitamin C need to look no further than the papaya. Long a folk remedy for allergies, indigestion and other problems, the fruit is rich in vitamin C. In fact, one raw papaya contains about 190 mg of vitamin C, or three times the RDA! Papayas also have over half the RDA for vitamin A, in the form of carotene, as well as a small amount of calcium and other nutrients.

Whole Grains

Whole grains such as wheat, rye and barley are good sources of the B vitamins and the mineral zinc. Studies and case histories show that various B vitamins can be helpful in controlling some of the symptoms of arthritis. Here are some examples:

- *Vitamin B_{12}* has reportedly helped reduce the pain of both chronic and acute bursitis.

- *Niacin* can help improve joint mobility in osteoarthritis patients.

  A French study conducted before World War II reported that skin lesions of systemic lupus erythematosus lessened when patients were injected with a form of niacin called niacinamide. The lesions began improving within a day, reaching a peak of improvement within several days.

- *Vitamin B_6* reduced pain and improved performance in a study of patients with carpal tunnel syndrome.

Several studies suggest that the B vitamins may be helpful in relieving some of the symptoms of arthritis. Because whole grains are an excellent source of B vitamins, it makes sense that eating plenty of servings on a daily basis may help you battle the disease.

Oysters

Oysters are an excellent source of zinc: Six medium-sized oysters offer just about 125 mg of the mineral, which is well over the RDA. Low blood levels of zinc and other nutrients have been associated with the joint pain and stiffness of arthritis, and bringing these levels back to normal may help reduce symptoms. We don't know exactly how zinc works to fight arthritis. However, it is a part of many enzymes, plays a role in bone health, is necessary for the digestion and production of proteins, and helps keep the immune system healthy.

Added Plus: Weight Managment

Nine of these ten super foods — fish, apples, spinach (and other green leafy vegetables), carrots, papaya, cantaloupe, grapefruit (and other citrus fruits), garlic, and whole grains — help combat osteoarthritis in yet another way that is beneficial. They are relatively low in calories, and consuming a diet made up of primarily low-calorie foods can help you lose weight. If you're overweight, shedding those excess pounds is an excellent way to relieve many of the symptoms of osteoarthritis in your hips, knees, and other weight-bearing joints.

Chapter 23

Ten Crackerjack New Treatments

● ●

In This Chapter

▶ The new form of NSAID

▶ Two "devices" that can help your joints work smoothly again

▶ The transplanting of cartilage from one joint to another

▶ Why controlling nitric oxide may relieve your pain

● ●

*I*n the not-too-distant future, physicians may be able to diagnosis arthritis by looking at a map of the patient's genes and treat this ailment through subtle genetic manipulation. In fact, doctors may be able to prevent arthritis from striking in the first place by studying an infant's genetic code and tweaking it to ensure that the young one's joints never begin the process of deterioration.

We're certainly not there yet, but medical researchers have developed a host of new treatments. Some are modern twists on older therapies, others are entirely new ideas.

Cox-2 Inhibitors: "New and Improved" NSAIDs

Two new drugs have entered the arthritis marketplace with great fanfare: Celebrex and Vioxx.

They're both classified as COX-2 inhibitors, a new and improved type of NSAID (nonsteroidal anti-inflammatory drug) that doctors hope will provide the same relief, with fewer side effects.

As described in Chapter 7, the NSAIDs relieve inflammation by interfering with an enzyme called COX (cyclooxygenase). But it turns out that there are two of these COX enzymes. COX-1 helps keep the stomach healthy, while

COX-2 plays a role in the inflammation process. The standard NSAIDs inhibit both COXs, the "good" and the "bad." As a result, your arthritis symptoms might have felt better when you took an NSAID, but your stomach was likely worse. The new COX-2 inhibitors target only the "inflammatory" COX-2, leaving the "healthy stomach" COX-1 alone to do its job.

Early results are promising: The COX-2 inhibitors appear to work as well as the old NSAIDs, with fewer side effects. The drawback is that these new medicines are more expensive. And because they're so new, we can't say with certainty that some long-term side effects won't show themselves somewhere down the road.

Here's some information on the two new COX-2 inhibitors:

Celebrex: Its generic name is celecoxib. Celebrex is used to relieve the pain, inflammation, and stiffness of osteoarthritis and adult rheumatoid arthritis. Although designed to have fewer side effects than the standard NSAIDs, Celebrex may cause diarrhea, abdominal pain, indigestion, ulceration, bleeding, and perforation of the stomach or intestines and other problems.

Certain conditions, such as pregnancy, asthma and allergies (to sulfa antibiotics and certain oral anti-diabetic drugs) make it dangerous to take Celebrex. It may also be dangerous to use Celebrex while you're on other medications or if you have liver or kidney disease.

According to its manufacturer, Celebrex has been tested in over 50 clinical trials. The manufacturer also states that 200 mg per day should be enough for osteoarthritis patients; either 200 mg once a day or 100 mg twice a day.

Vioxx: Its generic name is rofecoxib. Vioxx is meant to relieve osteoarthritis pain and inflammation, as well as acute pain in adults and menstrual pain. Although designed to have fewer side effects than the standard NSAIDs, Vioxx may cause bleeding in the intestines, kidney problems, nausea, itching, and tenderness in the right upper portion of the abdomen. There may also be flu-like symptoms, headache, dizziness, diarrhea, heartburn, swelling of the legs and/or feet, fatigue, urinary tract infection, vomiting, and other problems.

Certain conditions — such as pregnancy, asthma, swelling of the throat and face or other allergic reactions, allergies (to sulfa antibiotics, certain oral anti-diabetic drugs, rofecoxib or other NSAIDs) — make it dangerous to take Vioxx. Taking Vioxx while you're other medications or if you have liver disease, kidney disease, heart failure, high blood pressure, or certain other ailments can also be dangerous.

According to the manufacturer, a single pill per day may be enough for most people.

Both Celebrex and Vioxx are significantly more expensive than standard NSAIDs, costing between $90 and $120 per month. They're also relatively new, so the sum total of their effects, both good and bad, is not yet known.

Hyaluronic Acid Replacement for Osteoarthritis of the Knee

We normally picture bones when thinking of joints: two bones meeting and moving against each other. We often forget that such joints are "wet," bathed in a fluid that acts as both a shock absorber and lubricant, allowing joints to withstand the impact of movement and the bearing of weight, while the bones glide smoothly over each other.

Of course, not just any fluid will do; it must have certain properties and contain certain substances, including hyaluronic acid. A natural substance found not only in and around the joints but throughout the body, hyaluronic acid helps make the joint fluid viscous and able to absorb shock. It's also known as the "cement substance" of tissues and forms a gel between the cells.

If the joint fluid fails to do its job, it may be due to a lack of hyaluronic acid. But thanks to modern science, we can ask the doctor to "fill 'er up" by giving us injections of substances that function in much the same way, although they are only effective when used for osteoarthritis of the knee. There are two similar substances that can act as substitutes for missing or inadequate hyaluronic acid — Hyalgan and Synvisc. Both are injected directly into the joint, and their effectiveness and side effects are almost identical. The major difference between the two is the number of injections necessary: five shots for Hyalgan, three for Synvisc.

The jury is still out on these two devices (technically speaking they're medical devices, not drugs, because they are substituting for a substance normally found in the body rather than exerting a pharmacological action). Both performed well in studies, but not everyone responds to them so the medical community hasn't yet fully embraced them. One reason may be the cost: hundreds of dollars for either of these substances, plus the doctor's fee.

Hyalgan and Synvisc are given to patients suffering from mild to severe osteoarthritis of one or both knees who have not been helped by standard medications, physical therapy, exercise, or other modalities. They seem to work best in cases of mild to moderate osteoarthritis.

So far, reported side effects have been relatively few, including pain, swelling, redness, and other reactions in the joint where the substance was injected, including allergic reactions, rapid pulse, shivering, and fever.

Controlling TNF to Relieve Rheumatoid Arthritis

The immune system turns on the body in rheumatoid arthritis, which is one reason why drugs to suppress the immune system are used to control this disease. But that's a rather broad approach, one that interferes with the immune system's helpful actions as well as its harmful ones.

A new class of drugs has been devised to address that problem by focusing on very specific parts of the immune system, trying to spare the "good" parts of the immune response while stifling the "bad" ones. Called *biologic agents*, these drugs specifically interfere with the activity of TNF (tumor necrosis factor), a substance that plays a role in the inflammation process.

One of these biologic agents, Enbrel (generic name etanercept) is designed for people with moderate to severe rheumatoid arthritis who haven't been helped by standard disease-modifying medicines. Injected just beneath the skin twice weekly, Enbrel helps the body regulate TNF. In studies, a little over 60 percent of patients enjoyed a 20 percent or greater improvement in joint pain, joint swelling, and other criteria. The medicine works fairly quickly, so many patients were able to handle daily chores with greater ease within two weeks.

Enbrel is costly and has some potentially serious side effects. Some patients who were apparently prone to infections developed deadly infections while taking Enbrel. Other side effects included reactions at the injection site and headaches.

A drug called Remicade (generic name infliximab) is also designed to reduce the symptoms of rheumatoid arthritis by helping the body keep TNF under control. Originally used for Crohn's Disease, it was recently approved for patients with rheumatoid arthritis who have not responded well to the standard medications. Side effects of the drug, which is given intravenously once a month or once every two months, include infection of the upper respiratory tract, nausea, rash, cough, headache, fever, chills, chest pain, and changes in blood pressure.

Nitric Oxide Blockers for Inflammatory Arthritis

For years, nitroglycerin has been used to treat chest pain due to coronary artery disease. When patients feel the pain coming on, they quickly take a pill and usually start to feel better right away.

Nitroglycerin causes the body to release more nitric oxide (NO), which helps the blood vessels relax. It also helps fight infection and disease. But while we need NO, too much of a good thing can be bad. Overproduction of NO can worsen inflammatory conditions such as lupus and rheumatoid arthritis. During the inflammation process, release of excess NO can harm bodily tissues, including joints. The unfortunate result may be permanent tissue damage.

Researches are in the process of developing drugs that will help control NO levels in the body and the joint damage they cause. These drugs will not only help relieve symptoms but also prevent further tissue damage. Although drugs that control NO are not yet available to the public, clinical trials will be getting underway soon.

Prosorba for Severe Rheumatoid Arthritis

Prosorba isn't a drug. Instead, it's a device that "cleans" the blood in a process similar to kidney dialysis. The goal is to filter out certain antibodies in an attempt to calm an immune system that has turned on the body.

Designed for patients with severe rheumatoid arthritis who have not been helped by standard medications, Prosorba therapy requires 12 weekly sessions, each lasting about two hours. During the sessions, blood is taken from the arm, the fluid (plasma) and blood cells are separated, and the fluid is passed through a Prosorba cylinder. Inside the cylinder, the blood is filtered to remove the offending antibodies. Then the fluid and blood are combined before being returned to the body, via the other arm.

Not all patients are helped by Prosorba therapy, although 30 to 40 percent of those in clinical trials enjoyed good results, and some experienced remissions that lasted a year or longer. One thing is certain: It takes awhile to see results. On average it takes 9 to 12 weeks, and some people don't respond until they've undergone 16 to 20 weeks of treatment.

Unfortunately, Prosorba treatment is quite expensive, with each of the 9 to 20 sessions costing well over $1,000. And there are side effects, including nausea, muscle and joint pain, chills, fever, a temporary drop in blood pressure, and fatigue.

New DMARD to Help Control an Errant Immune System

A new disease modifying anti-rheumatic drug (DMARD) called Arava (leflunomide) attempts to reduce the symptoms of rheumatoid arthritis and the accompanying tissue damage by slowing the growth and reproduction of white blood cells. The rationale is that by interfering with white blood cells, which are involved in the inflammation process, joint pain and swelling is relieved, slowing the progression of tissue damage.

The first new DMARD to be approved by the government in a decade or more, Arava produces the same type of relief as does methotrexate, currently the most effective drug treatment for rheumatoid arthritis. But Arava has fewer and milder side effects than methotrexate, a cancer drug that can cause kidney failure and becomes less effective the longer it is used. Arava's side effects include possible liver problems, thinning or loss of hair, plus stomach and digestive problems. It may also cause birth defects and should be used with caution by women in their childbearing years. And Arava should be avoided if you have elevated blood pressure, problems with the immune system, kidney disease, and/or certain other conditions.

Arava doesn't cure rheumatoid arthritis, but it can help relieve symptoms and reduce the rate at which the disease progresses. It may also work for people who have not been helped by methotrexate or other medications, or those who can't tolerate methotrexate's side effects. If treatment with Arava is effective, patients can expect to see less joint swelling and tenderness in as little as four weeks.

Cartilage Self-Transplants

It would be nice if we could simply pop in a new "slab" of cartilage every time a joint went bad. Of course we can't, but doctors have figured out a way use healthy cartilage from a healthy joint to buff up a joint with cartilage that has seen better days.

The concept is simple: Use an arthroscope to take a small sample of cartilage from a healthy joint, "wash" this cartilage clean, and then let it grow and multiply in the laboratory. At the appropriate time, open up the damaged joint with an arthroscope and "plant" the cultured cartilage into the bad joint. If all goes well, the new, healthy cartilage will grow and multiply in the new location, replacing the diseased cartilage and restoring the damaged joint to health. And there's no problem with rejection because it's your very own tissue.

Cartilage self-transplantation is primarily performed on the knee. So far, the results are promising, with up to 80 percent of patients reporting improved joint function several months or years later.

Lyme Disease Vaccine

Researchers have developed a vaccine for Lyme disease that works in an unusual way. Instead of building the body's resistance to the disease before it strikes, the Lyme vaccine encourages the body to develop antibodies to a certain protein. Then, if you're bitten by an infected tick, that tick ingests the antibodies from your blood. Once inside the tick, the antibodies kill the *Borrelia burgdorferi* bacteria that cause Lyme disease. They kill the bacteria right in the tick's belly, *before* it can infect you. Pretty slick, isn't it?

While it's certainly an interesting idea, the Lyme vaccination is not necessarily the answer for everybody. Because it requires three injections over a 12-month period, it will probably only be used by people living in tick-infested areas. Also, a small number of immunized people have developed an autoimmune arthritis in reaction to the vaccine, and unfortunately, the vaccine isn't always effective.

Despite the drawbacks, you and your doctor may think it's worthwhile if you're often exposed to ticks that may be carrying the *Borrelia burgdorferi* bacteria.

"Resurfacing" the Ends of Bones

Although not yet available to the public, this resurfacing technique may soon ease pain in millions and millions of problem joints. The idea is simple: Coat the damaged bone ends with a polymer that "resurfaces" the area, allowing the bones to slide easily against each other, just as they did when the cartilage between them was healthy.

LPJ-394 to Reduce Lupus Flares

In December 1999, the results of an 18-month double-blind, placebo-controlled test with an experimental drug for lupus called LJP 394 were released. For a certain group of patients, the drug had been found effective at reducing the number of renal flares (episodes of kidney trouble), as well as lowering the necessary amounts of certain medications (corticosteroids and cyclophosphamide). Compared to people taking a placebo, the ones who used LJP 394 had less than half the number of renal flares.

The drug only worked for certain patients, and it's still experimental. But if more tests bear out these early promising results, LJP 394 may soon be helping other lupus patients.

Additional Supplements

There's scientific or anecdotal evidence that a lengthy list of other supplements can help combat arthritis, including:

- ✔ *DMSO (dimethyl sulfoxide):* DMSO is used abroad for rheumatoid and osteoarthritis, and in this country by veterinarians treating animals with musculoskeletal problems. There is some evidence indicating that DMSO helps relieve arthritis pain and stiffness, as well as the finger ulcers seen in scleroderma. Although it comes in a variety of forms, only medical-quality DMSO is appropriate for use in arthritis treatment.

- ✔ *MSM (methyl sulfonyl methane):* MSM is a sulfur-containing substance produced during the breakdown of DMSO. A number of animal studies, plus numerous case reports, suggest that it may help relieve inflammation. There are no generally accepted dosages for MSM, which comes in capsule and lotion form.

- ✔ *DHEA (dehydroepiandrosterone):* Levels of this substance are low in some people suffering form lupus, rheumatoid arthritis, and juvenile rheumatoid arthritis, suggesting that supplementation may be helpful. Early evidence is promising, and this mild male hormone naturally produced in the body may someday become an important weapon against arthritis. It's available in supplement form. An often-suggested dose is up to 200 mg per day.

- ✔ *Melatonin:* A hormone produced by the body, melatonin is a popular remedy for insomnia. A few studies suggest that it may be helpful in relieving some of the symptoms of fibromyalgia. An often-suggested dose is 1 to 3 mg per day, before bedtime.

✔ ***Green tea:*** Long considered to be helpful in staving off cancer, heart disease, and other ailments, green tea contains health-enhancing substances called catechins and polyphenols. It's plentiful supply of nutrients and powerful antioxidants may make it valuable for those with various forms of arthritis, and some animal studies point to its potential value in combating rheumatoid arthritis. Green tea comes "loose" and in tea bags, as well as in capsules. Some experts suggest drinking four or more cups of green tea every day, or getting the equivalent amount of catechins in supplement form.

✔ ***Magnesium:*** You can find this common mineral in many one-a-day supplements. It's certainly necessary for strong bones, and various studies suggest that it can help relieve some symptoms of fibromyalgia. Magnesium is found in wheat bran, wheat germ, almonds, cashews, brewer's yeast, buckwheat, peanuts, millet, whole grains, and tofu, among other foods. An often-suggested dose is up to 600 mg of magnesium daily.

✔ ***Bromelain***: An enzyme found in pineapple, bromelain is often used as a digestive aid because it can help break down protein. Bromelain also has anti-inflammatory properties that may help reduce the swelling and pain of arthritis. It comes in capsule form, and an often-suggested dose is 400 to 600 mg per day, three times a day.

Part VI
Appendixes

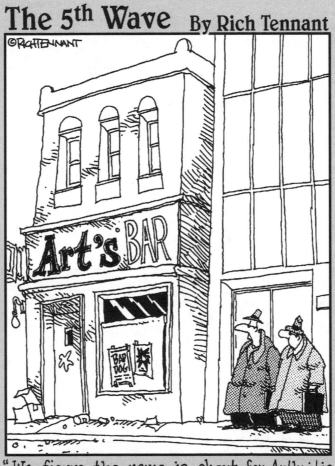

The 5th Wave   By Rich Tennant

"We figure the name is short for Arthritis because it's such a painful joint to have around you."

In this part . . .

For your convenience, included is a Glossary containing the most frequently used terms. You'll probably encounter these terms as you read information and talk to others about arthritis.

Appendix B is a list of resources. A lot of good, free information can be found on the Web as well, so we've listed Web sites whenever possible.

Appendix A

Glossary

· ·

Acupressure (Shiatsu): A Japanese form of massage that aims to restore health by normalizing the flow of energy and blood in the body.

Acupuncture: A part of Traditional Chinese Medicine that uses the insertion of very fine needles to help balance the flow of energy in the body.

Acute pain: Pain that typically strikes severely and suddenly, builds, then fades away. It occurs in response to injury, inflammation, surgery, and so on, and usually doesn't last long.

Alternative medicine: Healing techniques that fall outside of the realm of conventional, Western medicine.

Ankylosing spondylitis: A disease that causes inflammation and stiffness of the spine and its joints and that can result in the fusing or "locking" of those joints.

Antioxidants: Substances manufactured by the body and found in foods and supplements that help control the oxidation and free radical activity that can damage body tissue and cause or worsen certain disease states.

Aromatherapy: An alternative healing system based on the belief that inhaling certain aromas or scents can help the body heal itself.

Arthritis: A group of diseases (formerly called "rheumatism") that strikes the joints and/or nearby tissues. The word arthritis means "joint inflammation," although not all forms of arthritis cause inflammation.

Arthrodesis: Surgically immobilizing a joint so that the bones grow together and "lock" into position. This procedure is sometimes performed in cases of rheumatoid arthritis.

Arthroplasty: Surgical reconstruction of a joint using a combination of natural tissues and artificial parts; most commonly performed on the hip and knee.

Arthroscopy: Visual examination of the inside of a joint performed by using a special "scope" that is passed through a small incision. Arthroscopy can be used to diagnose certain types of joint disease and in some cases, make repairs surgically.

Autologous chondrocyte implantation: The transplantation of healthy cartilage cells from a normal joint to a damaged one, so that they can grow and supplement or replace ailing cartilage.

Ayurvedic healing: An ancient Indian healing art that uses diet, exercise, internal cleansing, herbs, massage, crystals, aromatherapy, color therapy, gems, and other modalities to eliminate illness and restore balance to the body.

Bee venom therapy: The use of bee venom to relieve pain and inflammation. The venom may be delivered via the sting of a live bee or through an injection.

Biofeedback: A method for helping one learn to exert some control over certain physiological functions, such as muscle tension or blood pressure. During a biofeedback session, you're hooked up to a machine that provides audio and visual feedback, as for example, muscle tension increases or decreases. Feedback from the machines shows you how certain body functions change as you relax.

Biomechanics: In a non-technical sense, it is the study of the way the body deals with its own weight — for example, the impact of walking or running on the weight-bearing joints. Using proper biomechanical techniques, one can greatly minimize the stress placed on the joints while moving, lifting, or even sitting.

Borrelia burgdorferi: The bacteria that causes Lyme disease, transmitted to humans by infected tick.

Bursitis: A painful condition resulting from inflammation of the bursae, the fluid-filled pouches that keep certain joints moving smoothly. Shoulder joints are likely targets of bursitis.

Calcium pyrophosphate dihydrate crystals: Crystals that can accumulate in a joint and cause the symptoms of pseudogout.

Capsaicin: The "hot" part of chili peppers. Capsaicin fights pain by stimulating nerve cells to release large amounts of substance P, which sensitizes the receptors that originate the pain signals. When the cells run out of substance P, pain signals subside.

Carpal tunnel syndrome: A condition caused by pressure on the median nerve as it runs through the "carpal tunnel," a narrow opening between the ligaments and bones in the wrist. Symptoms include pain, weakness, tingling, burning, and muscle atrophy.

Cartilage: Connective tissue found in the joints and elsewhere in the body. Joint cartilage helps protect bone ends that would otherwise rub against each other and produce pain and other problems.

Chinese medicine, traditional: An ancient healing art that seeks to cure disease by restoring body balance and ensuring that life energy (chi) flows freely throughout the body. Nutrition, herbs, acupuncture and other modalities are used.

Chiropractic: A healing system based on the belief that disease arises when spinal vertebrae are out of alignment and press on nerves. Chiropractic healing techniques include spinal manipulation and possibly exercise, nutrition, massage, and other modalities.

Chondroitin sulfate: A supplement that studies suggest can relieve symptoms of osteoarthritis. Often used in conjunction with glucosamine, chondroitin sulfate helps pull water into the cartilage and fight cartilage-eating enzymes that can damage this precious tissue.

Chronic pain: Pain that lasts weeks or months, that accompanies long-term disease, or that keeps recurring. It may continue long after the apparent cause has disappeared, and can significantly reduce the quality of life.

Color therapy: The use of color (in the form of light, clothing, food, gems, and so on) to help the body heal itself.

Complementary medicine: Non-standard healing approaches designed to work with conventional Western medicine.

Corticosteroids: A group of hormones naturally produced by the body that have wide ranging effects on metabolism, water balance, and organ function. The man-made versions have powerful anti-inflammatory properties but also have some serious side effects.

COX-2 Inhibitors: A relatively new form of NSAID with the same pain-relieving and anti-inflammatory benefits as other NSAIDs, but fewer side effects.

Deep tissue massage: The application of strong pressure to the muscles using fingers, hands, or elbows to relieve chronic tension in the muscles.

Dermatomyositis: A disease that produces muscle pain plus skin rashes and other problems.

DHEA (dehydroepiandrosterone): A hormone that the body uses to make testosterone, estrogen, and other hormones, and is sometimes used by alternative healers to treat lupus and other ailments. Sometimes called the "mother" of all hormones, it is produced primarily in the adrenal glands.

Discoid lupus erythematosus: A "limited" form of lupus that may produce a rash and other skin problems, weakening of the immune system, and other symptoms, but is not as severe as systemic lupus erythematosus.

DMARDs: Disease-modifying, antirheumatic drugs used for rheumatoid arthritis, psoriatic arthritis, and other forms of the disease. DMARDs appear to work by altering the behavior of the immune system.

DMSO (dimethyl sulfoxide): A form of alternative therapy, DMSO is a clear liquid that may be applied to the skin, injected, or swallowed in hopes of reducing arthritis pain and inflammation.

Fibromyalgia: A disease characterized by inflammation of the connective tissue, including the ligaments, tendons, and muscles. Symptoms include chronic achy pain, stiffness, disturbed sleep, depression, and fatigue.

Folk medicine: A body of non-standard remedies devised throughout history by people all over the world. Folk remedies include everything from eating chicken soup to ease congestion due to a cold to wearing a bandana soaked in vinegar wrapped around your head to relieve a headache.

Glucosamine: A supplement that studies suggest can relieve symptoms of osteoarthritis. Often used in conjunction with chondroitin sulfate, glucosamine is used by the body to manufacture proteoglycans, which draw water into the cartilage and keep it moist.

Gonococcal arthritis: The most common form of infectious arthritis, caused by the *gonococci* bacterium.

Gout: A type of arthritis caused by an accumulation of uric acid crystals in the joint, often the "bunion" joint of the large toe. Symptoms of gout include terrible pain, joint stiffness and swelling, and possibly fever, chills, and an elevated heart rate.

Herbalism (phytotherapy): The use of the roots, bark, stems, flowers, or other parts of selected plants to relieve the symptoms of illness and/or strengthen the body.

Holistic medicine: An approach to healing and health based on treating a patient's mind, body and spirit, rather than simply trying to counteract the disease or relieve symptoms.

Homeopathy: An alternative healing system developed in the eighteenth century, based on the belief that "like cures like." Thus, for example, patients suffering from nausea would be treated with very small doses of a substance that can cause nausea when given in large amounts to healthy people.

Hydrotherapy: The use of water, both hot and cold or in the form of steam, ice, compresses, and so on to relieve symptoms and help the body heal itself.

Immunosuppressants: Drugs that dampen the immune system. These may be used to treat rheumatoid arthritis, lupus, and other diseases in which the immune system is malfunctioning.

Infectious arthritis: Arthritis that is caused by the invasion of bacteria, viruses, or fungi.

Joint: The place where two bones meet. Joints can be moveable or fixed. There are gliding joints such as the spinal vertebrae, hinge joints such as the elbows, saddle joints such as the wrist, and ball-and-socket joints such as the hip.

Juvenile rheumatoid arthritis (JRA): The most common form of arthritis to strike children, producing pain or swelling in the joints, fever, anemia, and other symptoms.

Lyme disease: A disease caused by the *borrelia burgdorferi* bacteria, which is transmitted to humans through the bite of an infected tick. Lyme disease can produce a large "bull's eye" shaped rash at the bite site, swelling and pain in the joints, fever, fatigue, muscle aches, nausea, swollen lymph nodes, and other symptoms.

MSM (methyl sulfonyl methane): A breakdown product of DMSO, MSM is an anti-inflammatory used by some alternative practitioners to treat arthritis.

Myofascial release: A less painful form of Rolfing using gentle, steady pressure on muscle and fascia to ease pain and release tension.

Naturopathy: A healing art based on the belief that all diseases have natural causes and that the body has very strong, natural healing powers. Naturopathic physicians use diet, herbs, exercise, stress reduction, acupressure, and other modalities to help increase the body's healing prowess.

NSAIDs: Nonsteroidal anti-inflammatory medications designed to reduce pain and inflammation, often prescribed for various forms of arthritis.

Occupational therapist: A licensed professional who can help you cope with the day-to-day problems of living with arthritis (and other ailments) by finding easier ways for you to accomplish tasks, designing splints, recommending assertive devices, teaching you ways to protect your joints, and so on.

Omega-3 fatty acids: Sometimes called "fish oil" because their major source is certain types of fish, these substances can help reduce inflammation and other symptoms of rheumatoid arthritis, and possibly other forms of arthritis.

Orthopedist: A medical doctor specializing in diagnosing and treating problems of the bones, joints, muscles, and related tissues.

Osteoarthritis: A type of arthritis caused by the breakdown of cartilage, most often in the hips, knees, and other weight-bearing joints. Osteoarthritis may be due to injury, obesity, metabolic errors, heredity, or other factors.

Osteotomy: A surgical procedure during which a piece of bone is removed to improve joint alignment. It is sometimes used to treat osteoarthritis or ankylosing spondylitis.

Paget's Disease: A disease in which the body inappropriately breaks down and rebuilds bone, resulting in weaker bones, bone deformity, and other problems. Many Paget's patients are middle aged or older.

Physical therapy: The use of massage, exercise, hydrotherapy, electrical stimulation, and other modalities to help relieve pain, increase range of motion, strengthen muscles, and stimulate healing.

Polarity therapy: An alternative healing art based on the idea that the body contains "energy systems" that must be kept in balance. Polarity therapists attempt to find and release energy blockages by touching specific points on the body, and sometimes use gentle massage.

Polymyalgia rheumatica: A rheumatic condition characterized by severe, sudden stiffness in major joints, plus headaches, difficulty swallowing, coughing, and other symptoms.

Polymyositis: A disease producing inflammation of the muscles and loss of strength. There may also be joint pain, weight loss, Raynaud's phenomenon, and other symptoms. Polymyositis is like dermatomyositis, without the skin problems.

Pseudogout: A from of arthritis similar to gout, but caused by the accumulation of calcium pyrophosphate dihydrate crystals (rather than uric acid crystals) in the affected joint.

Psoriatic arthritis: Striking about 5 percent of those who have the skin condition known as psoriasis, psoriatic arthritis can cause inflammation, swelling, and sometimes joint deformity.

Raynaud's disease/phenomenon: A disease in which arterial spasms cause pain, burning, tingling, numbness, and/or discoloration, primarily in the fingers and toes. Raynaud's disease is more the common and often milder form; Raynaud's phenomenon is triggered by another ailment, such as lupus or scleroderma.

Reflexology: An alternative healing system based on the idea that specific areas of the feet are linked to parts of the body. Manipulating the point on the foot corresponding to the lungs, for example, is believed to help relieve some of the symptoms of asthma.

Reiki: A Japanese healing art in which the practitioner channels energy into the patient (often without touching) to help restore the flow and balance of energy in the body.

Reiter's syndrome: A disease that may develop after an infection. Reiter's can produce mild to severe pain in the joints, inflammation of the eyelid, eyeball and urethra, and other problems.

Rheumatoid arthritis: The second most common form of arthritis, rheumatoid arthritis is brought about when the immune system attacks the body. The result can be joint pain and inflammation, generalized soreness and stiffness, fever, difficulty sleeping, and joint deterioration. The disease can also attack the lungs, blood vessels, and other parts of the body.

Rheumatoid factor (RF): An antibody found in some 80 percent of those with rheumatoid arthritis. Its presence strongly suggests that one has rheumatoid arthritis, although it's possible to have RF and not develop the disease.

Rolfing: A technique developed in the 1950's based on the belief that body alignment affects mental, physical, and emotional health. To correct improper body alignment, the Rolfing practitioner stretches and manipulates the fascia covering bones, muscles, organs, and so on.

SAMe (S-adenosyl-l-methione): A product of body metabolism, SAMe is sometimes used in supplement form to combat depression and the symptoms of osteoarthritis.

Scleroderma: An autoimmune disease in which the body produces and stores excess collagen, resulting in damage to the skin, joint pain and swelling, difficulty swallowing, digestive difficulties, injury to the blood vessels, and damaged organs.

Sjögren's syndrome: A disease that produces dryness of the eyes and mouth and certain other parts of the body. Depending on the extent of the dryness and which parts of the body are affected, problems can range from the manageable to the very serious. A fair number of those with Sjögren's syndrome also develop arthritis, but this arthritis is most often a separate entity.

Soft tissue rheumatism: An old term indicating inflammation or pain in the bursae, tendons, ligaments, and other tissues surrounding and/or supporting the joints. Carpal tunnel syndrome is an example of soft tissue rheumatism.

Swedish massage: The gentle kneading and stroking of muscles, connective tissue, and skin to relieve stress and soothe pained muscles.

Synovectomy: A surgery in which an overgrown, inflamed joint lining is removed; it may be performed for rheumatoid arthritis.

Synovial membrane: Part of the capsule surrounding certain joints, this membrane releases a lubricating fluid into the joint.

Systemic lupus erythematosus: An autoimmune disease that "prefers" to attack women of child-bearing age. Systemic lupus erythematosus can cause a variety of symptoms, including joint pain and inflammation, fever, rash, hair loss, anemia, weakness of the immune system, depression, and nervous system disorders. It can be fatal.

Tendinitis: Inflammation of a tendon, characterized by pain to the touch or upon movement. The upper arms, hands, fingers, and backs of the ankles are common targets of tendinitis.

TENS: Transcutaneous Electrical Nerve Stimulation — the use of mild electrical currents to deliver small "jolts" to painful areas of the body. The electricity "overrides" pain signals.

Trigger finger: The locking of a finger in a bent position caused by swelling and inflammation of a tendon.

Trigger point therapy: Prolonged, deep tissue pressure applied to specific, tender and hard points on muscles to relieve tension and pain. The therapy may include injections of local anesthetic into trigger points.

Uric acid crystals: The offending agents in gout that accumulate in the joint, causing pain and other symptoms.

Urethritis: An inflammation of the urethra, the "tube" urine passes through to get from the bladder to the outside of the body.

Vasodilators: Medications that "relax" blood vessels and help blood flow more freely.

Resources

● ●

Organizations

Acupuncture/ Acupressure

Traditional Acupuncture Institute, American City Building,

10227 Wincopin Circle
Suite 100
Columbia, MD 21044-3422
Phone 301-596-3675 or 410-997-4888
E-mail: webmaster@tai.edu
Web site: www.tai.edu

American Academy of Medical Acupuncture

5820 Wilshire Blvd.
Suite 500
Los Angeles, CA 90036
Phone 800-521-2262
Web site: www.medicalacupuncture.org

National Certification Commission for Acupuncture and Oriental Medicine (NCCAOM)

11 Canal Center Plaza, Suite 330
Alexandria, VA 22314
Phone 703-548-9004
Web site: www.nccaom.org

Alexander Technique

American Society for the Alexander Technique

401 East Market Street
Charlottesville, VA 22902
Phone 800-473-0620
E-mail: nastat@ix.netcom.com
Web site: www.alexandertech.org

Alexander Technique International

1692 Massachusetts Avenue, Third Floor
Cambridge, MA 01238
Phone 888-321-0856
E-mail: usa@ati-net.com

Alternative Medicine

National Center for Complementary & Alternative Medicine (NCCAM) Clearinghouse

P.O. Box 8218
Silver Spring, MD 20907-8218
Phone 888-644-6226
Web site: http:altmed.od.nih.gov/hccam

Aromatherapy

National Association for Holistic Aromatherapy (NAHA)

P.O. Box 17622
Boulder, CO 80308
Phone 303-258-3791
Web site: www.naha.org

Pacific Institute of Aromatherapy

P.O. Box 6842
San Rafael, CA 94903
Phone 415-479-9121

Arthritis Information and Management

Arthritis Foundation

1330 West Peachtree Street
Atlanta, GA 30309
Phone 800-283-7800 or 404-872-7100
or call your local chapter
Web site: www.arthritis.org

American College of Rheumatology

1800 Century Place, Suite 250
Atlanta, GA 30345
Phone 404-633-3777
E-mail: acr@rheumatology.org
Web site: www.rheumatology.org

American Juvenile Arthritis Organization

1330 West Peachtree Street
Atlanta, GA 30309
Phone 404-965-7514
E-mail: ajao@arthritis.org
Web site: www.arthritis.org/answers/
children_young_adults.asp

Fibromyalgia Network

P.O. Box 31750
Tucson, AZ 85751-1750
Phone 800-853-2929
Web site: www.fmnetnews.com

Lupus Foundation of America, Inc.

1300 Piccard Drive, Suite 200
Rockville, MD 20850
Phone 800-558-0121 or 301-670-9292
Web site: www.lupus.org

Myositis Association of America

755 Cantrell Avenue, Suite C
Harrisonburg, VA 22801
Phone 540-433-7686
Web site: www.myositis.org

National Institute of Arthritis, Musculoskeletal and Skin Diseases (NIAMS) Information Clearinghouse

1 AMS Circle
Bethesda, MD 20892-3675
Phone 877-226-4267 (toll free) or 301-495-4484
Web site: www.nih.gov/niams

The Paget Foundation

120 Wall Street, Suite 1602
New York, NY 10005
Phone 212-509-5335
E-mail: pagetfdn@aol.com
Web site: www.paget.org

The National Psoriasis Foundation

6600 SW 92nd Avenue, Suite 300
Portland, OR 97223
Phone 503-244-7404
E-mail: getinfo@npfusa.org
Web site: www.psoriasis.org

The Scleroderma Foundation

89 Newbury Street, Suite 201
Danvers, MA 01923
Phone 800-722-4673 or 978-750-4499
E-mail: sfinfo@scleroderma.org
Web site: www.scleroderma.org

Sjogren's Syndrome Foundation

366 No. Broadway
Jericho, NY 11753
Phone 800-475-6473
Web site: www.sjogrens.org

Spondylitis Association of America (SAA)

14827 Ventura Blvd., Suite 222
P.O. Box 5872
Sherman Oaks, CA 91413
Phone 800-777-8189 or 818-981-1616
E-mail: info@spondylitis.org
Web site: www.spondylitis.org

Ayurvedic Medicine

National Institute of Ayurvedic Medicine

584 Miltown Road
Brewster, NY 10509
Phone 888-246-6426
E-mail: drgerson@erols.com
Web site: www.niam.com

The Ayurvedic Institute

11311 Menaul NE
Albuquerque, NM 87112
Phone 505-291-9698
Web site: www.ayurveda.com

The American School of Ayurvedic Sciences

2115 112th Avenue NE
Bellevue, WA 98004
Phone 425-453-8022
E-mail: ayurveda@ayush.com
Web site: www.ayurvedicscience.com

Bee Venom Therapy

American Apitherapy Society

5390 Grande Road
Hillsboro, OH 45133
Phone 937-364-1108
E-mail: aasoffice@in-touch.net
Web site: www.apitherapy.org

Biofeedback

The Association for Applied Psychophysiology and Biofeedback

10200 W. 44th Ave., Suite 304
Wheat Ridge, CO 80033
Phone 800-477-8892 or 303-422-8436
Web site: www.aapb.org

Biofeedback Certification Institute of America

10200 W. 44th Ave., Suite 304
Wheat Ridge, CO 80033
Phone 303-420-2902
Web site: www.bcia.org

Biomechanics Experts

American Academy of Osteopathy

3500 DePauw Blvd., #1080
Indianapolis, Indiana 46268
Phone 317-879-1881
Web site: www.academyofosteopathy.org

Chiropractors

American Chiropractic Association (ACA)

1701 Clarendon Blvd.
Arlington, VA 22209
Phone 800-986-4636 or 703-276-8800
Web site: www.amerchiro.org

ChiroWeb – Everything chiropractic for chiropractors, students, patients and health care consumers

Web site: www.chiroweb.com

DMSO/MSM

Dr. Stanley Jacob, DMSO Research Institute

L225, 3181 S.W. Sam Jackson Park Road
Portland, OR 97201-3098
Phone 503-494-8474
E-mail: jmueller@dmso.org
Web site: www.dmso.org

Feldenkrais Method

The Feldenkrais Guild of North America (FGNA)

524 Ellsworth Street SW
Albany, OR 97321-0143
Phone 800-775-2118
E-mail: feldngld@peak.org
Web site: www.feldenkrais.com

Help for Caregivers

Family Caregiver Alliance

690 Market Street, Suite 600
San Francisco, CA 94104
Phone 415-434-3388
E-mail: info@caregiver.org
Web site: www.caregiver.org

National Family Caregivers Association

10400 Connecticut Avenue, #500
Kensington, MD 20895-3944
Phone 800-896-3650
E-mail: info@nfcacares.org
Web site: www.nfcacares.org

Homeopathic Medicine

National Center for Homeopathy

801 N. Fairfax St.
Suite 306
Alexandria, VA 22314
Phone 703-548-7790
Web site: www.homeopathic.org

Homeopathic Educational Services

2124B Kittridge St.
Berkeley, CA 94704
Phone 800-359-9051 or 510-649-0294
E-mail: mail@homeopathic.com
Web site: www.homeopathic.com

Hypnotherapists

American Council of Hypnotist Examiners (ACHE)

700 So. Central Avenue
Glendale, CA 91204-2011
Phone 818-242-1159
Web site: www.sonic.net/hypno/ache.html

National Guild of Hypnotists

P.O. Box 308
Merrimack, NH 03054-0308
Phone 603-429-9438
E-mail: ngh@ngh.net

Massage Therapists

The American Massage Therapy Association

820 Davis Street, Suite 100
Evanston, IL 60201
Phone 847-864-0123
E-mail: info@inet.amtamassage.org
Web site: www.amtamassage.org

Associated Bodywork & Massage Professionals

1271 Sugarbush Drive
Evergreen, CO 80439-7347
Phone 800-458-2267 or 303-674-8478
E-mail: expectmore@abmp
Web site: www.abmp.com

National Certification Board for Therapeutic Massage and Body Work

8201 Greensboro Dr., Suite 300
Mclean, VA 22102
Phone 800-296-0664
E-mail: mswiscoski@ncbtmb.org
Web site: www.ncbtmb.com

Medical Societies

American Academy of Orthopaedic Surgeons

6300 North River Road, Suite 200
Rosemont, IL 60018-4262
Phone 800-346-2267 or 847-823-7186
Web site: www.aaos.org

American Academy of Physical Medicine and Rehabilitation

One IBM Plaza, Suite 2500
Chicago, IL 60611-3604
Phone 312-464-9700
Web site: www.aapmr.org

American Board of Medical Specialties

1007 Church St., Suite 404
Evanston, IL 60210-5913
Phone 847-491-9091
Web site: www.abms.org
(Can provide you with referrals to physicians who are board-certified in orthopedic surgery, pain management, rheumatology, surgery, and other specialties.)

American Board of Surgery

1617 John F. Kennedy Blvd.
Suite 860
Philadelphia, PA 19103-1847
Phone 215-568-4000
Web site: www.absurgery.org

American Medical Association

515 N. State St.
Chicago, IL 60610-4320
Phone 800-621-8335 or 312-464-5000
Web site: www.ama-assn.org

American Occupational Therapy Association

4720 Montgomery Lane
P.O. Box 31220
Bethesda, MD 20824-1220
Phone 800-377-8555 or 301-652-2682
Web site: www.aota.org

American Physical Therapy Association

1111 N. Fairfax St.
Alexandria, VA 22314
Phone 703-684-2782
Web site: www.apta.org

The Mind/Body Connection

The Academy For Guided Imagery

P.O. Box 2070
Mill Valley, CA 94942
Phone 415-389-9324
Web site: www.interactiveimagery.com

The Mind-Body Medical Institute

Beth Israel Deaconess Medical Center,
Division of Behavioral Medicine
110 Francis Street
Suite 1A
Boston, MA 02215
Phone 617-632-9530
E-mail: mbmi@caregroup.harvard.edu
Web site: www.mindbody.harvard.edu

Naturopathic Medicine

The American Association of Naturopathic Physicians

601 Valley Street, Suite 105
Seattle, WA 98109
Phone 206-298-0126
E-mail: aanp@usa.net
Web site: www.naturopathic.org

Bastyr University

14500 Juanita Drive NE
Kenmore, WA 98028-4966
Phone 425-823-1300
Web site: www.bastyr.edu

The Homeopathic Academy of Naturopathic Physicians

12132 S.E. Foster Place
Portland, OR 97266
Phone 503-761-3298
E-mail: hanp@igc.apc.org
Web site: www.healthy.net/hanp

Pain Management

American Academy of Pain Management

13947 Mono Way, Suite A
Sonora, CA 95370
Phone 209-533-9744
Web site: www.aapainmanage.org

American Chronic Pain Association

P.O. Box 850
Rocklin, CA 95677
Phone 916-632-0922
E-mail: ACPA@pacbell.com
Web site: www.theacpa.org

American Pain Society

4700 West Lake Avenue
Glenview, IL 60025
Phone 847-375-4715
E-mail: info@ampainsoc.org
Web site: www.ampainsoc.org

Polarity Therapy

American Polarity Therapy Association

P.O. Box 19858
Boulder, CO 80308
Phone 303-545-2080
E-mail: hq@polaritytherapy.org
Web site: www.polaritytherapy.org
(Call or write to get a copy of the APTA
Members Index, which lists all members by
region. Cost is $3.00)

Psychotherapy

American Psychological Association

Office of Public Affairs
Washington, D.C. 20002-4242
Phone 202-336-5700
E-mail: public.affairs@apa.org

National Register of Health Service Providers in Psychology

1120 G Street, NW, #330
Washington, D.C. 20005
Phone 202-783-7663
Web site: www.nationalregister.com

American Association for Therapeutic Humor

222 So. Meramec, #303
St. Louis, MO 63105
Phone 314-863-6232
Web site: http://aath.org

Reiki

The International Center for Reiki Training

21421 Hilltop Street, Unit #28
Southfield, MI 48034
Phone 800-332-8112
E-mail: center@reiki.org
Web site: www.reiki.org
(see link: Reiki Net Resources)

Reflexology

Reflexology Association of America

4012 Rainbow Blvd.
Suite K
Box 585
Las Vegas, NV 89103-2059
Phone 702-871-9522
Web site: www.reflexology-usa.org

Support Groups Online

ArthritisWebSite.Com

Web site: www.arthritiswebsite.com
(click "Community Voice")

Support-Group.Com

Web site: www.Support-Group.com

National Mental Health Consumer Self-Help Clearinghouse

1211 Chestnut Street, #1207
Philadelphia, PA
Phone 800-553-4539 or 215-751-1810
Web site: www.mhselfhelp.org
(For information about how to start your own self-help group.)

Therapeutic Touch

Nurse Healers – Professional Associates International (The Official Organization of Therapeutic Touch)

11250-8 Roger Bacon Drive, Suite 8
Reston, VA 20190
Phone 703-234-4149
E-mail: nhpai@drohanmgmt.com
Web site: www.therapeutic-touch.org

Trager Approach

The Trager Institute

21 Locust Avenue
Mill Valley, CA 94941-2806
Phone 415-388-2688
E-mail: admin@trager.com
Web site: www.trager.com

Assistive Devices — Mail Order Catalogs

adaptAbility: Products for Quality Living

75 Mill St., P.O. Box 515
Colchester, CT 06415-0515
Phone 800-288-9941

Dr. Leonard's Healthcare Products

100 Nixon Lane
P.O. Box 7821
Edison, NJ 08818-7821
Phone 800-785-0880

Don Kreb's Access to Recreation: Adaptive Recreation Equipment

P.O. Box 5072-430
Thousand Oaks, CA 91362
Phone 800-634-4351

IMAK Products Corporation (ergonomic products)

2918 Fifth Avenue 200
San Diego, CA 92103
Phone 800-231-8226
E-mail: customercare@imakproducts.com

Independent Living Aids, Inc. Can-Do

27 East Mall
Plainview, NY 11803
Phone 800-537-2118

InteliHealth HealthyHome

97 Commerce Way
P.O. Box 7007
Dover, DE 19903
Phone 800-988-1127

Life With Ease (ergonomic products)

P.O. Box 302
1329 Route 103
Newbury, NH 03255
Phone 603-763-7339
E-mail: contact@lifewithease.com

Maxi-Aids and Appliances for Independent Living

P.O. Box 3209
Farmingdale, NY 11735
Phone 800-522-6294 or 516-752-0521

North Coast Medical AfterTherapy Catalog

Distributed by Access to Recreation, Inc.
2509 East Thousand Oaks Blvd., Suite 430
Thousand Oaks, CA 91362
Phone 800-634-4351

PHS West, Inc. (motorized carts)

11283 River Road NE
Hanover, MN 55341
Phone 612-498-7576
E-mail: phsw@uswest.net

Sammons Preston Enrichments

P.O. Box 5071
Bolingbrook, IL 50440-5071
Phone 800-323-5547
Web site: www.sammonspreston.com

SoftFLEX Computer Gloves

4230 Winding Willow Drive
Tampa, FL 33624
Phone 800-216-8414
E-mail: sales@softflex.com

Books

Arthritis Helpbook: What You Can Do For Your Arthritis, 3rd Ed. Lorig, K. and Fries, J.F. Reading Massachusetts: Addison-Wesley, 1990. Call Addison-Wesley at (800) 447-2226.

Eighty-Eight Easy-To-Make Aids for Older People and for Special Needs. Caston, D., Point Roberts, WA: Hartley and Marks, Inc., 1988. Call Hartley and Marks at (206) 945-2017.

Guide to Independent Living for People With Arthritis. Arthritis Foundation. Available at your local Arthritis Foundation chapter or write to Bulk Order Department, Arthritis Foundation, 1314 Spring Street NW, Atlanta, GA 30309.

Help Yourself: Recipes and Resources From the Arthritis Foundation. Available at your local Arthritis Foundation chapter or call (800) 283-7800.

The Illustrated Directory of Handicapped Products. Behzad, M.S., Ed., Lawrence, K.S.: Trio Publications, Inc. Write to Trio Publications at 3600 West Timber Court, Lawrence, KS 66049.

Raising A Child With Arthritis: A Parent's Guide. Arthritis Foundation. Available at your local Arthritis Foundation chapter or call (800) 283-7800.

250 Tips For Making Life With Arthritis Easier. Arthritis Foundation. Available at your local Arthritis Foundation chapter or call (800) 283-7800.

Videos

These videos are available at your local Arthritis Foundation chapter or call (800) 283-7800:

People with Arthritis Can Exercise (PACE) I. Basic strengthening, stretching and cardio-fitness exercises to help you tone up and regain your range of movement.

People with Arthritis Can Exercise (PACE) II. A more advanced version of PACE I, with the same goals in mind.

Pool Exercise Program (PEP). By exercising in water (no deeper than chest level) you can get a great workout while putting little or no strain on your joints.

Pathways to Better Living With Arthritis. Using gentle exercises and techniques borrowed from yoga such as deep, rhythmic breathing, stretching and relaxation, you can get excellent results while really enjoying your workout.

Weight Loss and Management Guide

• •

*E*ven if you're eating a balanced, "pyramidal" diet, getting plenty of omega-3s, and avoiding danger foods, there's one more step to take — the one that puts you up on a scale. And if what you see when you look at the dial doesn't look good, it's time to lose weight.

If you're overweight or obese, one of the best things you can do for your aching joints is to lose weight. Cutting away the extra pounds takes a tremendous burden off those joints that have to bear your weight, such as your hip and knee joints. Not only does it take the pressure off, there's strong evidence that dropping down to your ideal weight can stave off the appearance of at least one form of arthritis.

The Framingham Study used X rays to track the development of arthritis in women. The researchers found that the women who had dropped 5 pounds before the X rays were taken, that is, before the "zero" point, were only about half as likely to develop the disease as the women who had held their weight steady or gained. And a study sponsored by the Arthritis Foundation found that older and overweight women could lower their risk of developing osteoarthritis of the knee – significantly – by reducing their weight.

How Do You Know If You're Too Heavy?

On average, adult Americans have packed on an additional eight pounds in the past decade, and we're continuing to grow. Medical experts agree that it's better to be slim, especially where arthritis is concerned. But what's slim? Unfortunately, we're not very good at knowing when enough is enough. In general, women tend to think they're too heavy, and men usually assume they're doing okay — "nothing a few trips to the gym couldn't fix."

For years, we've looked at height-weight charts to see if we should drop a few pounds, but they were only rough guidelines. In 1998, a division of the National Institutes of Health issued a new set of guidelines based on the body mass index (BMI), a comparison of height and weight. Now you just look for one number, your BMI, too see if you need to lose weight. Here are the standards:

- ✔ If your BMI is 24 or less, you're fine.
- ✔ If it's between 24 and 29, you're overweight. Those extra pounds are beginning to challenge your health and put extra pressure on your joints.
- ✔ If it's over 30 you're obese. Your weight is or likely will cause health problems.

So you want your BMI to be no more than 24, and certainly less than 29. The formula for determining BMI is simple: Multiply your weight in pounds by 703 and divide the answer by your height in inches squared. Well, maybe it's not so simple. Table C-1 will help you skip the figuring and get a fairly good idea of where you stand.

Table C-1	Body Mass Index Chart		
Height	Weight That Gives a Healthy BMI of 24	Weight That Puts You in the Overweight BMI Range	Weight That Gives an Obese BMI of 30
5'0"	123	124-153	154
5'1"	127	128-158	159
5'2"	131	132-163	164
5'3"	135	136-168	169
5'4"	140	141-174	175
5'5"	144	145-179	180
5'6"	149	150-185	186
5'7"	153	154-191	192
5'8"	158	159-196	197
5'9"	162	163-202	203
5'10"	167	167-208	209
5'11"	172	173-214	215
6'0"	177	178-220	221
6'1"	182	283-226	227
6'2"	187	187-233	234

The BMI is not an absolutely perfect guide to weight. It only compares height to weight, it doesn't take into account that fact that some people appear "fatter" and get higher BMIs because they have lots of muscles. For others, the reverse can be true because they don't have a lot of muscle. Still, it's a good starting point.

Losing Weight the Safe and Healthy Way

The bad news is that there's no such thing as a quick, simple, guaranteed way to lose weight. The gimmicks don't work; the fad diets don't live up to their promises. Oh yes, you'll lose weight on most any fad diet, primarily because they all get you to restrict your intake one way or another. And many of them cause you to quickly lose lots of water weight. But most people quickly gain back all the water weight — and all the other weight as well. The overwhelming majority of people who drop pounds on fad diets gain them back — plus a few more. And to make matters worse, a fair number of fad diets are nutritionally unbalanced: Eating what they recommend for long periods of time can lead to trouble.

The good news is that it is possible to lose weight without sacrificing nutrition or health. We can't go into great detail on losing weight, because this isn't a diet book. Fortunately, there are many books presenting safe, sensible and effective diets, including *Dieting for Dummies* by the American Dietetic Association and Jane Kirby.

Most people already know how to lose weight. Notwithstanding the hype in the fad diet books, the basic principles for healthy people are simple: Eat a well-rounded diet emphasizing fresh vegetables, whole grains and fruits, keep your fat content down to reasonable levels, enjoy sweets as occasional treats, and burn lots of calories through physical activity and exercise. In short, burn more calories than you take in.

A plan for long-term benefits

Don't diet. "Dieting" is a bad word, it means giving up favorite foods and eating a lot of stuff you don't like, or starving yourself. It's a short-term fix to be discarded as soon as possible.

Instead, eat for lifelong good health. Focus on the slow, steady and permanent weight loss that comes when your diet and activity/exercise habits are in alignment.

Eating fruits and vegetables is always right

Eat a variety of vegetables, fruits and whole grains to ensure that you get all the numerous nutrients in foods. No single food or food group gives you all you need, for there's no such thing as a "magic" food. Eat less meat, poultry and dairy products, but when you do, eat many different kinds.

Limiting your intake of certain foods

Take it easy on cholesterol, saturated fat, sugar and salt.

Eat sweets sparingly. Many people have found that the more they cut back, the less they crave these foods. Don't look upon it as depriving yourself: Just cut back a little bit at a time. You may be surprised to find that your desire falls off with your consumption.

Read the labels on your food cans and packages carefully. You'd be surprised at how many calories food makers squeeze into some foods you thought were fairly "lite."

Psychological strategies to get you through

Put smaller portions on your plate. That way you can "clean your plate" without stuffing yourself.

Avoid places and settings that normally cue to you overeat. For example, if you always gobble down plates and plates of fried chips and gooey, fatty cheese dip when you meet your friends at the Mexican restaurant for an after-work drink, try going somewhere else.

Don't shop when you're hungry, for the growl in your stomach will tempt you to buy sweets and fattening foods.

Set a reasonable goal. Don't try to lose 30 pounds a month, or squeeze into that teensy bathing suit by next week. People who lose weight that fast usually put it back on, almost as rapidly. If you stick to a good eating/exercise plan and only lose a quarter or a half pound a week, that's fine.

Don't be too hard on yourself if you don't meet all your goals exactly on schedule. You're only human; you're allowed some leeway. And besides, you're eating for life; you're in it for the long haul. You don't have to sprint, but just stay on the right track.

When you do something great, reward yourself with something other than food.

It's not just what you eat . . .

Remember that what you do or do not eat is only half the equation. You must also burn up calories with physical activity and exercise.

Eat slowly. It takes a while for your brain to catch up with what you're eating, so it's possible to eat more than you want or need if you shovel it in. Take your time, let your brain register the fact that you've eaten. You'll eat less that way.

"Pre-eat" a little bit before going to parties, movies and other places where you can't get healthful food. If you eat a small portion of health-enhancing food before you go out, you won't be tempted to overdo the popcorn and chocolate once you're there. Instead, you can enjoy a little, as a special treat.

Eyeballing those portions

Many diets suggest specific portion sizes, such as 3 oz. of fish or ½ cup of vegetables or 8 oz. of milk. But because few of us carry little food scales or measuring cups, we're often forced to estimate. Eyeball estimations can be difficult because most people tend to underestimate the portion size of foods they enjoy eating and over estimate those they don't like. (Ever notice how a ½ cup of ice cream looks like nothing, but a ½ cup of beets looks like way too much?)

Table C-2 offers some tips developed by Sheldon Margen and Dale Ogar for eyeballing food portion sizes. The tips are easy to remember, or if you like, you can cut the table out and carry it in your wallet or pocketbook.

Table C-2	Visual Food Portion Guidelines
Quantity	*Visual Aid*
How big is a 3 oz. serving?	About the size of a deck of cards.
What's 1 serving of pancake or waffle?	A pancake or waffle the size of a 4-inch CD.
How much is a 1 teaspoonful?	About the size of the tip of your thumb.
What's a ½ cup serving of veggies, rice, pasta or cereal?	Cooked, a mound about the same size as a small fist (or baseball).
How big is a small baked potato?	Roughly the size of a computer mouse.
What's a medium apple or orange?	One about the size of a baseball.
What's an ounce of cheese?	About the size of four dice.

Index

• F •

• *G* •

Notes

Notes

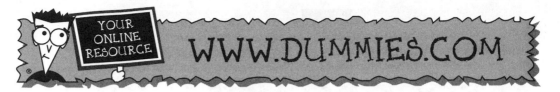

Discover Dummies Online!

The Dummies Web Site is your fun and friendly online resource for the latest information about *For Dummies*® books and your favorite topics. The Web site is the place to communicate with us, exchange ideas with other *For Dummies* readers, chat with authors, and have fun!

Ten Fun and Useful Things You Can Do at www.dummies.com

1. Win free *For Dummies* books and more!
2. Register your book and be entered in a prize drawing.
3. Meet your favorite authors through the IDG Books Worldwide Author Chat Series.
4. Exchange helpful information with other *For Dummies* readers.
5. Discover other great *For Dummies* books you must have!
6. Purchase Dummieswear® exclusively from our Web site.
7. Buy *For Dummies* books online.
8. Talk to us. Make comments, ask questions, get answers!
9. Download free software.
10. Find additional useful resources from authors.

Link directly to these ten fun and useful things at **http://www.dummies.com/10useful**

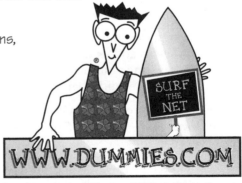

For other technology titles from IDG Books Worldwide, go to www.idgbooks.com

Not on the Web yet? It's easy to get started with *Dummies 101*®: *The Internet For Windows*® *98* or *The Internet For Dummies*® at local retailers everywhere.

Find other *For Dummies* books on these topics:

Business • Career • Databases • Food & Beverage • Games • Gardening • Graphics • Hardware
Health & Fitness • Internet and the World Wide Web • Networking • Office Suites
Operating Systems • Personal Finance • Pets • Programming • Recreation • Sports
Spreadsheets • Teacher Resources • Test Prep • Word Processing

IDG BOOKS WORLDWIDE BOOK REGISTRATION

Register This Book and Win!

We want to hear from you!

Visit **http://my2cents.dummies.com** to register this book and tell us how you liked it!

- ✔ Get entered in our monthly prize giveaway.

- ✔ Give us feedback about this book — tell us what you like best, what you like least, or maybe what you'd like to ask the author and us to change!

- ✔ Let us know any other *For Dummies®* topics that interest you.

Your feedback helps us determine what books to publish, tells us what coverage to add as we revise our books, and lets us know whether we're meeting your needs as a *For Dummies* reader. You're our most valuable resource, and what you have to say is important to us!

Not on the Web yet? It's easy to get started with *Dummies 101®: The Internet For Windows® 98* or *The Internet For Dummies®* at local retailers everywhere.

Or let us know what you think by sending us a letter at the following address:

For Dummies Book Registration
Dummies Press
10475 Crosspoint Blvd.
Indianapolis, IN 46256

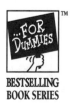

FOR DUMMIES™

BESTSELLING BOOK SERIES